Clinical Anthropology 2.0

Anthropology of Well-Being

Individual, Community, Society

***Series Editor*:** Ben G. Blount, PhD (SocioEcological Informatics)

Mission Statement

Well-being is central and important in people's daily lives and life history. This book series brings about understanding of what the complex concepts of well-being include. The concepts of quality of life, life satisfaction, and happiness will be explored and viewed at the individual level, the community level, and the level of society. The series encourages and promotes research into the concept of well-being, how it appears to be defined culturally, and how it is utilized across levels and across different social, economic, and ethnic groups. Understandings of how well-being promotes stability and resilience will also be critical to advances in understanding, as well as how well-being can be implemented as a goal in resisting vulnerabilities and in adaptation. Series books include monographs and edited collections by a range of academics, from rising scholars to experts in relevant fields.

Advisory Board Members

Steven Jacob, Kathleen Galvin, Carlos Garcia-Quijano, Cynthia Isenhour, and Richard Pollnac

Recent Titles in the Series

Clinical Anthropology 2.0: Improving Medical Education and Patient Experience, by Jason W. Wilson and Roberta D. Baer

Living with HIV in Post-Crisis Times: Beyond the Endgame, edited by David A.B. Murray

Diversity and Cultural Competence in the Health Sector: Ebola-Affected Countries in West Africa, by Mohamed Kanu, Elizabeth A. Williams, Charles Williams, and Regina Bash-Taqi

Everyday Food Practices: Commercialisation and Consumption in the Periphery of the Global North, by Tarunna Sebastian

No Perfect Birth: Trauma and Obstetric Care in the Rural United States, by Kristin Haltinner

Love and its Entanglements among the Enxet of Paraguay: Social and Kinship Relations within a Market Economy, by Stephen Kidd

Clinical Anthropology 2.0

Improving Medical Education and Patient Experience

Jason W. Wilson and Roberta D. Baer

LEXINGTON BOOKS
Lanham • Boulder • New York • London

Published by Lexington Books
An imprint of The Rowman & Littlefield Publishing Group, Inc.
4501 Forbes Boulevard, Suite 200, Lanham, Maryland 20706
www.rowman.com

86-90 Paul Street, London EC2A 4NE

Copyright © 2022 by The Rowman & Littlefield Publishing Group, Inc.

All rights reserved. No part of this book may be reproduced in any form or by any electronic or mechanical means, including information storage and retrieval systems, without written permission from the publisher, except by a reviewer who may quote passages in a review.

British Library Cataloguing in Publication Information Available

Library of Congress Cataloging-in-Publication Data

Names: Wilson, Jason W., 1978- author. | Baer, Roberta Dale, author.
Title: Clinical anthropology 2.0 : improving medical education and patient experience / Jason W. Wilson and Roberta D. Baer.
Description: Lanham, Maryland : Lexington Books, 2022. | Series: Anthropology of well-being | Includes bibliographical references and index.
Identifiers: LCCN 2021051713 (print) | LCCN 2021051714 (ebook) | ISBN 9781498597685 (cloth) | ISBN 9781498597708 (paperback) | ISBN 9781498597692 (ebook)
Subjects: LCSH: Medical anthropology. | Medical anthropology—Study and teaching. | Public health—Anthropological aspects. | Medical education. | Physician and patient.
Classification: LCC GN296 .W556 2022 (print) | LCC GN296 (ebook) | DDC 306.4/61—dc23/eng/20211201
LC record available at https://lccn.loc.gov/2021051713
LC ebook record available at https://lccn.loc.gov/2021051714

We dedicate this book to all of the physicians, and graduate, medical, and premedical students with whom we have worked over the years. And we look forward, in the coming years, to their authorship of Clinical Anthropology 3.0. We also acknowledge and appreciate our patients at Tampa General Hospital who have shared their experiences, and taught us so much about the human condition.

Contents

Acknowledgments

We thank all those at the University of South Florida and at Tampa General Hospital who have supported our work.

Chapter 1

Introduction

In this book we detail our work, and that of our students, in one of the most challenging environments for a medical anthropologist: an urban hospital. We begin from the perspective that applied medical anthropology in such a context is not an example of "selling out to the neoliberal system," but rather a context in which we can do research which directly contributes to some of the key problems patients face in medical settings. All anthropology has colonial origins, and many academic disciplines must both confront and reflect on those pasts while assembling new ways forward. Rylko-Bauer, Merrill Singer, and John Van Willigan (2006) do an excellent job considering prior criticisms of applied work and dismiss the notion that applied anthropology is somehow more prone to neoliberal and colonial pressures than other areas of the field, while also making clear that praxis is not mutually exclusive to theory (2006).

Our project began by introducing premedical undergraduates to a Level 1 trauma center—the Emergency Department (ED) of Tampa General Hospital (TGH)—and has now expanded into other parts of the hospital (outpatient primary care system, inpatient hospital units, and mobile healthcare stations all associated with TGH). After beginning our work with premedical undergraduates, we have expanded to include medicine faculty, internal medicine residents, and medical students. In addition, we have further solidified the relationship between the ED, the hospital, and an academic applied anthropology department at the University of South Florida (USF) by placing graduate students into clinical spaces at the urban hospital to complete PhD and MA level projects, as well as to move forward research and operations through a funded postdoctoral position.

Our graduate students are often embedded within the hospital for multiple years and work directly with physicians, healthcare teams, students, and medical residents. We believe that an anthropological lens sheds light and creates unrecognized pathways for patients that were previously unseen. Contemporary issues and patient populations which we have explored include firearm injuries, the opioid epidemic, the development of a structurally competent approach to patient care, recognition of social determinants in healthcare, pain management in patients with sickle cell disease, the Covid-19 pandemic, high utilizers of healthcare services, physician-patient communication, as well as physician satisfaction scores that attempt to measure the patient experience and are related to provider and institution reimbursement.

In all of this, our approach has been shaped by multiple anthropological perspectives. Arthur Kleinman's perspective, described by him, Eisenberg, and Byron Good in 1978 has been key; the perspective that patients and providers have different models is as relevant today as it was over 40 years ago. If anything, the gap between patient illness presentation and the provider approach has widened as providers must meet multiple obligations during a patient encounter not only to the patient but also to the biomedical system (billing, quality, compliance). Our students—even medical residents in the middle of their rigorous clinical training—remain shocked to discover how modern this reading still seems over 40 years after publication. Hahn's (1996) further discussions of the distinct culture of biomedicine are also still important, as are the cases which Chrisman collected in his 1982 book, *Clinically Applied Anthropology*.

We move beyond the latter, however, as its focus was specifically on the way that medical care can improve to be more responsive to the needs of patients. We also discuss how the contributions of our perspective can contribute to the fit between physician expectations and the actual patient needs and issues with which medical staff are confronted (e.g., opioid dependence which is more prevalent than acute heart attacks in many ED populations); it is this mismatch which we feel contributes to physician burnout. We also advocate for a role expanded over that which Chrisman discusses (1982) and feel that the clinically applied medical anthropologist should become one of the actors in the healthcare setting, not merely an observer of it. And the focus is not only the patients but also the larger system of care. Further, we do not limit the role of the anthropologist to situations where the patient is of a non-mainstream cultural background. Instead, we follow Kleinman et al. (1982) and Hahn (1996), defining each medical encounter as a cross-cultural experience between the patient, the provider, and the healthcare system while also recognizing that structural forces determine much of the variability between patient encounter types and outcomes. These patient encounters reproduce and reify structural barriers, widen gaps between patients and providers, and make it impossible to define static cultural concepts or to create models for "cultural competency" (Cigna Inc., Website).

Our key approach to teaching dates to Malinowski as we emphasize the importance of participant observation, but for the purposes of our work, we have renamed this as patient shadowing (both using the common nomenclature in medicine and seeking buy-in among students to actively engage in the heuristic activity). In the chapters below we detail how the use of this technique in the medical setting can quickly produce changes in perspective not only for undergraduate premedical students but also for medical students, as well as medical residents.

The chapters in this book outline our work to date in this setting. Chapter 1 introduces the focus of the book. Chapter 2 develops the theoretical underpinnings of our approaches, which are clearly linked to anthropology and applied anthropology. In chapter 3 we discuss our first project, taking undergraduate premedical students to the ED and having this setting serve as a research base for class projects. Such a class is not without challenges, and these are addressed in chapter 4. Chapter 5 discusses the ways we have expanded into training of medical personnel at other levels, such as second-year internal medicine residents at TGH and first-year medical students at the USF Morsani College of Medicine.

Chapters 6 to 10 address contributions to Quality Improvement and new patient pathways in clinical settings, focusing on the projects we have developed and continue to develop as we expand and apply our ideas regarding the role of medical anthropology in the clinical space. While our initial work focused significantly on the education of physicians and future physicians (chapters 3 to 5), we do fully recognize that much of the clinical gaze must be shifted not only by education but also by participatory action as part of interdisciplinary teams. Those teams should include medical anthropologists working in the clinical space.

In chapters 6 to 10, we discuss clinical studies and interventions which have incorporated medical anthropological perspectives and methodologies directly in the ED, hospital, and other clinical areas. These projects also demonstrate models of education and training for future medical anthropologists doing applied work with clinical healthcare teams. In chapter 6 the leaflet project is addressed. The creation of a patient leaflet began as a class project and now involves hospital-wide personnel working together to produce a patient-centered informational leaflet for use in the ED. Chapter 7 details work with multi-visit patients, whose high use of ED services poses a challenge. Chapters 8 ("Sickle Cell Disease"), 9 ("Language, Pain, and Nontraditional Patient Treatment Spaces"), and 10 ("Opioids and Infectious Disease") involve work with some of the populations which are most challenging to Emergency Medicine (EM) personnel. Often these populations of patients are felt to require increased time for management and have fewer clear pathways established for disease management. Many EM providers do not feel well trained to address these specific types of populations, which we refer to as "special populations in the ED," that is, those that have illness for which formal organic disease is not as well understood or studied. These populations have historically led to provider frustration during the patient encounter, perhaps magnifying physician burnout or leading to poor patient experiences measured by decreased patient satisfaction scores. Much of this work has also been done with graduate students in the USF Applied Anthropology Program who have worked with us in the ED.

The projects described in these chapters vary in focus, but all these projects encompass anthropological methods to generate new approaches to challenging healthcare problems. The projects differ in the type of medical anthropological involvement, from premedical students doing a class project, to undergraduate anthropology students and honors students individually investing more time into specific project areas, to an MA student working over two years in the ED to develop approaches to patients with limited English proficiency and, most formally, the work of a PhD student and postdoc fellow now doing work on opioid use disorder and infectious disease.

In these chapters, we discuss the overall chapter content, a conceptual and literature review of the specific issue, the type of medical anthropological involvement (e.g., student, level of training), the methods, findings, and what contribution the work has made to the ED or hospital. We demonstrate how increasingly complex projects can be undertaken in clinical settings by incorporating medical anthropology education or by integrating more trained medical anthropologists. Finally, each chapter details the anthropological difference—the unique contributions that were possible because of the engagement of medical anthropology methods, theory, and people.

Finally in chapter 11, we show an expansion of our approaches to include new ways to investigate contemporary public health concerns. We discuss one of our projects which began in the undergraduate course—our study of the broad consequences of firearm violence for those who survive these injuries. Using qualitative interviews, we explore the medical and social consequences of such injuries and consider these patients' perspectives on firearm policies.

All this work is shaped by our conviction that applied medical anthropology has underrecognized role in the biomedical healthcare system. In the past, applied medical anthropologists have served roles just outside of the clinical encounter. In contrast, we believe a clinically applied medical anthropologist brings high value inside the clinical space by providing the lens to recognize structural determinants of healthcare and the recognition of provider, patient, healthcare system cultures. We believe that applied medical anthropologists should contribute to medical personnel training and that this enriched training would lead to improved patient experiences and, potentially, decreased levels of physician burnout by better equipping providers with the tools to manage disease as well as illness (Kleinman et al. 1978). In addition, we strongly feel that the gap between disease and illness and the frustration with repeat patient visits for seemingly non-biomedical complaints can be minimized by medical anthropologists working directly in the clinical space to create a linkage between patient and provider perspectives. This will help to demonstrate the existence and needs of otherwise hidden, unseen, or stigmatized "special populations." Our experiences demonstrate how such programs, rooted in medical anthropology, can be successful and have a direct impact in clinical settings.

Chapter 2

Can There Be a Critical, Clinically Applied Medical Anthropology?

In this chapter, we outline the theoretical perspectives in medical anthropology that have influenced our approaches: clinically applied anthropology (Chrisman and Maretzki 1982), critical medical anthropology (CMA) (Singer and Baer 1985; Farmer 2006; Ortner 2016), and applied anthropology (Ervin 200). We propose a synthesis of these perspectives is most appropriate for framing the work we are doing. Parallel to these developments, we review changes in approaches to biomedicine, as well as other recent attempts to link anthropology and medicine, many of which have been proposed by a new generation of physician anthropologists (e.g., Kim Sue, Seth Holmes, Scott Stonington, Eugene Richardson).

CLINICALLY APPLIED ANTHROPOLOGY

This approach to medical anthropology is synthesized in the work of Chrisman and Maretzki (1982). Their edited volume, Clinically Applied Anthropology, reviewed the work of anthropologists in health science settings. It focused on the approaches used by these anthropologists to address clinical issues related to health maintenance and response to sickness. Contributors described their successful projects to justify their presence in such settings. A key concern was to make healthcare more responsive to the needs of patients and the need to promote humanistic rather than veterinary standards in medical care (Young 1981).

However, clinically applied approaches were narrow and came to focus primarily on finding ways to achieve patient compliance to biomedical treatment plans and to closing the gap between biomedical and cultural explanatory models of disease and illness. This approach may also have overfocused on psychiatric-related questions and cognitive theory.

CMA

CMA has become the dominant contemporary paradigm for analysis in the discipline of medical anthropology (Good 1992). Previous applied approaches emphasizing clinically important outcomes (clinically applied anthropology) were largely dismissed during the 1990s with the rise of critical theory (Scheper-Hughes 1990).

By the early 1990s, CMA questioned assumptions regarding human structure and power that were taken for granted or minimized when considering how culture drives and distributes variation in healthcare seeking and healthcare outcomes. Instead, upstream structure explained inequities between and across human groups. During that same period, there was growing recognition that anthropologists themselves may be blinded to, creators of, contributors or coconspirators with, those forces leading to human inequity, that is, a postmodern turn. Complicating developments in cultural theory further was a realization of epistemological variation that led to renewed interest in understanding how humans make and engage with meaning and knowledge production itself. While much of nineteenth- and twentieth-century anthropology was concerned with identifying, defining, and considering both the definition and function of culture, the late twentieth century and the new millennium saw a shift in interest to interhuman group dynamics and knowledge production with some focused on the politics of power and another set of scholars turning more inward toward philosophical considerations of meaning and epistemology.

Late twentieth-century shifts in anthropological theory led to a focus on asymmetric power between institutions and individuals. How these power structures are produced and reified became driving concerns that could be addressed theoretically and locally, not just by traveling to describe a far-off other. These questions also open a door, if not demand, for anthropological involvement in both local, if not broader, issues of social justice and advocacy.

This period also saw the rise of structural approaches as explanatory of differential healthcare access developed in medical anthropology with a focus on structural violence, found in Paul Farmer's work on tuberculosis, HIV, and other infectious disease distributions (Farmer 2003). However, some have been concerned that these structural approaches dismiss the role of culture (and reading Farmer's *Pathologies of Power* might accentuate that concern).

By 2016, cultural anthropology had moved past a focus on understanding culture, as anthropologists themselves, and the populations they studied, experienced the forces of change that come with the global neoliberalism (Ortner 2016). Within the context of growing recognition that essentially all human groups were subject to rapid change and socio-politically structured inequality, postmodern theory within the discipline led to the emphasized realization that anthropologists themselves brought their own identity to their work, objects of study, and their interpretations of human groups.

APPLIED ANTHROPOLOGY

Applied anthropology dates formally to the establishment of the Society for Applied Anthropology in 1941 (SfAA Website). But Erwin (2000) notes that some of the earliest "traditional" anthropology was done in applied contexts—including the work of British social anthropologists in colonial Africa. Applied anthropology continued to be important in the 1940s, during World War II, and afterward (Spicer 1952). However, the 1960s saw the expansion of academic employment for anthropologists and the beginning of the perspective that applied anthropologists were second class and ethnically challenged. However, this rosy job market soon evaporated. The year 1974 saw the development of the first applied anthropology graduate programs devoted to training practitioners. The movement has only expanded since, and currently, there are about 30 such programs in the United States.

Parallel to this, as discussed earlier, have been the developments of theoretical perspectives in anthropology and medical anthropology that have further stigmatized applied anthropology. Postmodernism has stressed the lack of one set of facts or truth, which makes the applied task of using ethnographic data to develop policy challenging. CMA accused practitioners of being part of a neoliberal hegemonic biomedicine (Scheper-Hughes 1990). The important focus of CMA on structure became an all-out attack on the concept of culture. Many applied anthropologists working in clinical settings became alienated from the main theorists in medical anthropology (see, for example, the work of Chrisman et al. 1999, Erwin 2008, Matthews 2014), even though the programs and policies they were developing precisely addressed the structural issues so appropriately emphasized by CMA.

Our work is committed to bringing these perspectives together. Patient-physician interactions cannot be understood without the concepts of explanatory models (Kleinman et al. 1978) and the distinct culture of biomedicine (Hahn 1996). We view every clinical interaction as a cross-cultural experience for all the participants. But structural constraints and structural violence are key to understanding why patients present for healthcare, where and when they do, and the extent to which they can comply with clinical recommendations.

DEVELOPMENTS IN MEDICINE

These theoretical perspectives from anthropology are encountering a new focus in medicine, concerned with evaluation of performance (and subsequent funding levels), based on patient satisfaction scores. In 2017, Tampa General Hospital (TGH) received another C rating on the national benchmark Leapfrog Patient Safety Report (Leapfrog Group, Website). In 2020, the rating finally moved from a C to a B; however, Doctor-Patient communication remained "below average." In addition, the Centers for Medicare and Medicaid Services (CMS) gave the institution a three-star rating (out of five) in 2020 (Star Rating Site, CMS). That improved to a four-star rating in 2021, after intensive efforts in the Emergency Department (ED) and across the hospital space to improve patient experiences.

Those who practice at TGH do not feel that they provide three-star, C level care to their patients—they think they provide excellent and innovative care on a world-class level. No one wakes up and goes to work thinking that they will only perform at a C level (whoops, left that sponge in there, forgot to wash my hands, ah, who needs antibiotics?). As physicians (JWW), most of us value the time we must spend and talk with patients, discussing their disease and illness, covering their treatment plans, outlining options for how to proceed next. So, what gives? Why do these physicians struggle to improve their ratings? (figure 2.1a, figure 2.1b).

A key issue is that there is a mismatch between why patients present to the ED, the training of physicians, the expectations of physicians, and the expectations of patients. As patient experience (measured through patient satisfaction scores) becomes increasingly important, this mismatch is magnified and worsened. Previously, physicians may have been able to overlook the demands and expectations of their patients who did not mesh with the physicians' perspectives of why patients should come to the ED and how patients should respond to treatment options. In a consumer-driven model of healthcare delivery, however, it is not acceptable or possible for physicians to structure an ED encounter to their own model of how the visit should go. Instead, the encounter must mutually unfold as a shared unraveling of why the patient came to the ED and how best the physician can help navigate differences in explanatory models of disease and illness.

Often, "illness" (Kleinman et al. 1978) is the primary reason for the patient visit and, if the physician is not better equipped to deal with the structural and cultural context of that illness, both the patient and physician will likely be frustrated. A self-perpetuating disintegrating cycle continues where the physician and patient both become angrier with each other and the medical system. This frustration will result in low patient satisfaction scores which impact both the physician's reimbursement and hospital funding.

	TAMPA GENERAL HOSPITAL	FLORIDA AVERAGE	NATIONAL AVERAGE
Patient survey summary star rating. More stars are better. Learn more	☆☆☆●●		
Patients who reported that their nurses "Always" communicated well	81%	77%	81%
Patients who reported that their doctors "Always" communicated well	79%	77%	82%
Patients who reported that they "Always" received help as soon as they wanted	64%	65%	70%
Patients who reported that staff "Always" explained about medicines before giving it to them	65%	62%	66%
Patients who reported that their room and bathroom were "Always" clean	72%	71%	76%
Patients who reported that the area around their room was "Always" quiet at night	61%	58%	62%
Patients who reported that YES, they were given information about what to do during their recovery at home	87%	84%	87%
Patients who "Strongly Agree" they understood their care when they left the hospital	57%	51%	53%
Patients who gave their hospital a rating of 9 or 10 on a scale from 0 (lowest) to 10 (highest)	78%	69%	73%
Patients who reported YES, they would definitely recommend the hospital	81%	70%	72%

Figure 2.1a Centers for Medicare and Medicaid Services (CMS) Hospital Compare Star Ratings. https://www.medicare.gov/care-compare/

Physicians recognize patterns, and types of patients are categorized based on thousands of physician-patient interactions. Future similar patients will generate frustration in the physician before they even see the patient. The patient is also concerned because they are seeking care from a physician in an environment where they have previous experiences that did not relieve suffering and perhaps only resulted in structural violence. It is structural because the act of violence is a designed part of the healthcare system, and violence because the delivery, or lack of delivery, of medical care causes further harm to a patient (as the concept is explained by Galtung, 1969 and discussed by

	TAMPA GENERAL HOSPITAL	FLORIDA AVERAGE	NATIONAL AVERAGE
Patient survey summary star rating. More stars are better. Learn more	☆☆☆●●		
Patients who reported that their nurses "Always" communicated well	81%	77%	81%
Patients who reported that their doctors "Always" communicated well	79%	77%	82%
Patients who reported that they "Always" received help as soon as they wanted	64%	65%	70%
Patients who reported that staff "Always" explained about medicines before giving it to them	65%	62%	66%
Patients who reported that their room and bathroom were "Always" clean	72%	71%	76%
Patients who reported that the area around their room was "Always" quiet at night	61%	58%	62%
Patients who reported that YES, they were given information about what to do during their recovery at home	87%	84%	87%
Patients who "Strongly Agree" they understood their care when they left the hospital	57%	51%	53%
Patients who gave their hospital a rating of 9 or 10 on a scale from 0 (lowest) to 10 (highest)	78%	69%	73%
Patients who reported YES, they would definitely recommend the hospital	81%	70%	72%

LEAPFROG
HOSPITAL
SAFETY GRADE

This Hospital's Grade

B

FALL 2019

Communication with doctors

Figure 2.1b 2019 Tampa General Hospital Leapfrog Ratings (Leapfrog 2019). *Source*: https://ratings.leapfroggroup.org/facility/details/88-6426/tampa-general-hospital-tampa-fl #return:facility=Tampa+General+Hospital&by=facility&sort=relevance.

Farmer, 2006). The patient, who may be placed in a hallway bed, may not receive access to a professional interpreter, may have several imaging and laboratory studies competed, and then may be discharged from the ED without a clear explanation of the patient's symptoms or suffering that caused them to originally seek care.

A Twitter exchange initiated by a community Emergency Medicine (EM) Physician exemplifies these expectation mismatches and the development of physician burnout and poor patient experiences.

According to the National Academy of Medicine (formally the Institute of Medicine), there is an ongoing epidemic of physician burnout in healthcare (NAM 2016). While physician wellness is now recognized as a driver of this burnout, how do we improve the situation? How do we close the gap between physician and patient expectations? If physicians are not able to match their expectations with patients—who comes to the ED and why?—the burnout epidemic is likely to continue and will be visible via poor satisfaction scores.

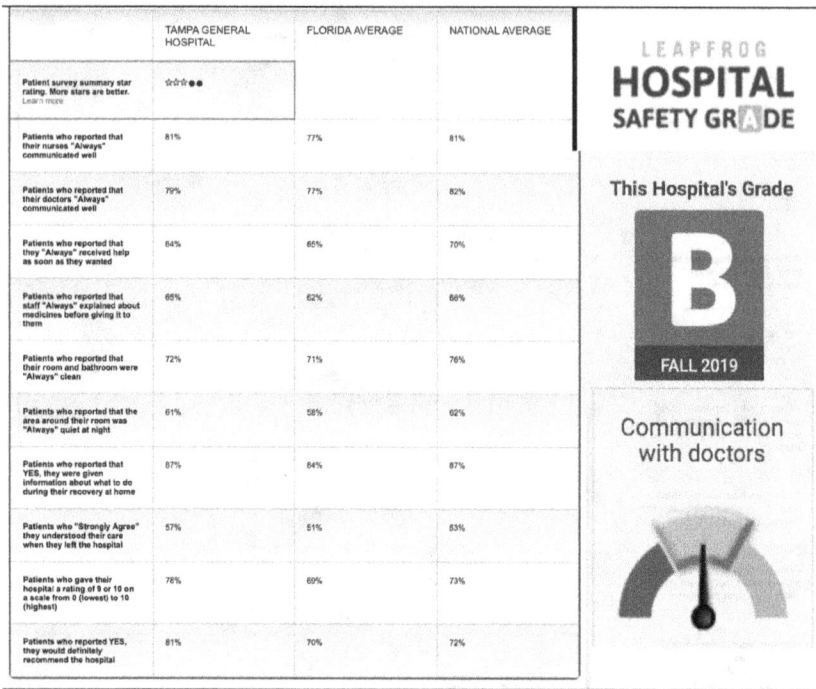

We hypothesize that many patients seeking care in the ED undergo everyday structural violence, largely secondary to explanatory model mismatch, that creates suffering. While EM physicians are trained to focus on pathophysiology of disease, it is structurally rooted pathways of suffering (financial inequity, power asymmetry, violence) that drive patients to seek care in the ED, creating a patient-physician mismatch. Explanatory models of disease and illness differ between physicians and patients, and that variability is often driven by cultural differences both between laypeople and providers (Kleinman et al. 1978, Hahn 1996), but also between different subpopulations due to structural factors.

Furthermore, physicians have developed their own burnout culture based on anger and frustration with their training that does not prepare them well for the types of patients that present to the ED, the hospital, or the clinic. This is because physicians have been trained to expect that ED patients will primarily be trauma and cardiac patient—in their eyes, "true" emergencies. The anger is increased when they are shown patient satisfaction scores highlighting areas needing improvement in the overall patient experience. The patient satisfaction scores eventually drive down reimbursement, lead to administrative criticism, and worsen the anger further, especially as more patients seek care for reasons that the physician does not consider acceptable for that specific clinical space (e.g., opioid dependence in the ED).

While limited in theoretical grounding, the motivation within medicine to directly impact patient encounters and the healthcare system is tangible. The Society of Academic Emergency Medicine (SAEM) has a Social Determinants and Population Health interest group (SAEM Website), with a nascent focus on praxis, that is still formulating its approach and purpose. Simultaneously, theory in medical anthropology has advanced to consider the role of structural forces in healthcare but, over the past few decades, has become more insular in approach and even hostile to interactions with biomedicine. This has the effect of, largely, leaving biomedical providers with a view of only knowing medical anthropology as a field that teaches methods of "cultural competence," seemingly only designed to overcome falsely static and stereotypical cultural identity patterns in a way to assimilate patients into desired treatment plans and pathways.

Unfortunately, many current approaches to cultural competence have done little more than reify such stereotypical understandings of cultural variation, grounded in analysis of the population as divided by the U.S. Census categories. Obviously, medical anthropology has more to offer healthcare than these simplistic notions of cultural competence. However, a new approach to clinically applied medical anthropology will be needed to synthesize disparate approaches to medicine and culture that have evolved within anthropology since the late 1980s when attempts to fully define a clinically applied approach were largely abandoned with the rise of CMA (Scheper-Hughes 1990).

Much of the gap in healthcare delivery exists within the inability to recognize processes and formations of new and emerging patient disease and illness, which challenge biomedical essentialism. In other words, biomedical teaching revolves around understanding of binary pathology categories of sick and not sick, or risk stratification of patients into biologically more likely to become sick or not sick. Reality has demonstrated that structural forces continually alter why patients get sick, how they get sick, and who comes to the ED. Current anthropological approaches to understanding and focusing on knowledge production and the process of formations open new ways that medical anthropologists could be utilized in clinical spaces.

Physicians are not just searching for ways to get patients to take their blood pressure medicine, but now, instead, are looking for ways to elevate the patient experience, ensuring that patient experience outcomes are linked appropriately to reimbursement. They are also concerned with, examination of where and when patients encounter the healthcare system, making sure the right patient goes to the right place at the right time, while also trying to manage a workforce that is increasingly diverse and fearful of rapid changes in the larger healthcare system.

In medicine, a larger shift to value-based purchasing and patient-centered high-quality care has been ushered in as part of the triple aim which includes patient experience, per capita cost, and experience of care (CMS Website). These are all elements that now drive system design and reimbursement strategies, thus placing increased focus on measurements of patient experience through patient satisfaction scores and increased scrutiny on the efficacy of healthcare interventions to provide meaningful improved patient outcomes. More recently, a move to recognize a healthcare staff burnout epidemic has also been encapsulated by some into this paradigm, expanding the triple aim to a quadruple aim approach (Bodenheimer and Sinsky 2014). The triple aim has envisioned an improved health system that simultaneously pursues the patient experience of care, the health of populations, and a reduction in cost. Bodenheimer and Sinsky (2014) go further and suggest that the triple aim is not achievable unless the healthcare workforce can find meaning and joy. Thus, a new landscape has emerged with a real opportunity for applied medical anthropology to help improve patient experiences.

This is because physicians do not have extensive training in approaches to culture, structure, or patient experience. As these domains have increased in priority over the past decade, a potential dissonance between physicians and healthcare has emerged that harkens back to explanatory model mismatches first outlined by Kleinman et al. (1978). Those mismatches, however, are not just between how patients and providers understand disease and illness, but instead are created by discordance between the distribution of illness for which patients seek care in an ED compared to the reasons physicians *think* patients should seek care in an ED. Deeper anthropological-based education models that begin to incorporate structural competency into medical curriculum can also help to decrease the expectation mismatch distance between what physicians think their jobs entail compared to what patients actually engage the healthcare system for and expect during an encounter.

PHYSICIAN ANTHROPOLOGISTS

As we are moving past outdated concepts of cultural competence as the main offering from anthropology to medicine, we are instead developing a notion of culture as a process of a meaning-making, occurring repeatedly during patient encounters that exist within the biomedical structure. If done correctly, a structural competency frame can be a more easily applied way for physicians to consider what they largely call the social determinants of health. While Chrisman et al. (1982), Kleinman et al. (1978), and Good (1992) mostly focused on one-on-one clinical patient encounters, a focus on structural violence and structural determinants has allowed a shift in broader healthcare system organizational injustices and asymmetries, widening the potential role and value of applied anthropologists.

Certainly, more nuance in the terms "cultural" and "structural competency" will be necessary if applied medical anthropology is to help develop contemporary clinical approaches. The involvement of applied medical anthropologists who have formal training in medicine and anthropology is an important pathway to connecting two disciplines while maintaining the reflexive approach that is still needed when working directly within the biomedical paradigm. Peter Brown has trained physician anthropologists (Salhi 2018, Salhi et al. 2018) and one of the authors (JWW), is simultaneously completing a PhD in anthropology while practicing as an EM physician, in addition to opening a research space for medical anthropology students to begin answering difficult biomedical questions using mixed methods approaches (see chapters 4 to 10)

In addition, Seth Holmes, Scott Stonington, Helena Hansen, and Paul Farmer, all physician-anthropologist, have initiated a series of case vignettes in the *New England Journal of Medicine* (2018) that consider structure and clinical practice. The case presentation approach is familiar to physicians, making unfamiliar theory and subject matter easier to consider in their own practice. Stonington et al. (2018) state,

> In their first year in medical school, all students learn to take a social history. As they transform their eyes, ears, and hands into sensors for detecting hidden causes of disease, they also learn to ask probing questions to illuminate patients'

> social contexts. What pathogenic exposures might a patient face en route to immigrate to the United States from Guatemala, in being subjected to police violence and arrest in a heavily patrolled nonwhite neighborhood, in working in pesticide-laden fields, or as a result of exclusion from health care coverage? Answers to such questions can dramatically change a diagnostic picture or therapeutic plan. Yet by the clinical years of medical school, students learn that the social history is often collapsed into a record of three biobehavioral exposures—to alcohol, tobacco, and illicit drugs. Much of what they read in clinical journals appears to corroborate the assumption that in clinical medicine, the biologic and behavioral world of a patient's body is more important than the social world outside it. (2018: 1958)

As the emphasis on social determinants (vs. individual behavior) decreases during the rapid paced work of clinical training, the realization that disease is explained, mostly, by structural forces more so than novel genetic markers, familial inheritance patterns, or in situ unexplained biological pathways also decreases among physicians in training. Physicians recognize that poverty, nutrition, and labor all explain disease distribution but, in the parlance of Foucault (1973), the clinical gaze is trained to assign individuality to these structural forces and to overplay the role of agency in "choosing" risk behaviors that lead to poor health outcomes (Foucault 1973). An attempt to shift the clinical gaze must be part of the clinically applied medical anthropology

Table 2.1 Key Questions for Disease/Illness (Kleinman et al. 1978) Compared to Hansen and Metzl (2016) in Seymour et al. (2018) Key Questions for Structural Competency.

Kleinman et al (1978)	Hansen and Metzl (2016), Seymour, Griffin, Holmes, Martinez (2018)
What do you think caused your problem?	Do you have enough money to live comfortably—pay rent, get food, pay utilities/telephone?
Why do you think it started when it did?	Do you have a safe, stable place to sleep and store your possessions?
What do you think your sickness does to you?	Do the places where you spend your time each day feel safe and healthy?
What are the chief problems your sickness has caused for you?	Do you have adequate nutrition and access to healthy food?
What do you fear most about your sickness?	Do you have friends, family, or other people who help you when you need it?
What kind of treatment do you think you should receive?	Do you have any legal problems?
What are the most important results you hope to get from the treatment?	Can you read?
	Have you experienced discrimination?
	*Authors also suggest asking yourself: May some service provider, including me, find it difficult to work with this patient?

approach. Structural approaches are most accessible to clinicians who, by definition, are concerned with praxis. These approaches allow an entry into considering social determinants of disease distribution, impacts on patient-level health outcomes, and can, ultimately, provide a pathway to consideration of cultural concepts of knowing, embodiment, deservingness, and suffering.

Physician-Anthropologist Helena Hansen and physician-sociologist Jonathan Metzl (2016) have proposed a structural competency curriculum for medical schools that focuses on patient-level encounters and offers concrete tools for students and practitioners to take to bedside. In addition, physician team Cheryl Seymour and Carrie Griffin, along with physician-anthropologist Seth Holmes and researcher Carlos Martinez, developed a five-question structural vulnerability guide (Seymour et al. 2018) like Kleinman's key questions (Kleinman et al. 1978) for the provider to assess differences in patient and physician explanatory models of illness and disease (Metzl and Hansen 2014). We outline these questions in table 2.1.

DIRECTIONS FORWARD

The focus of clinically applied anthropology in the 1980s is no longer relevant to modern medicine. And the narrow outsider focus of critical med anthropology has left out applied anthropology. In addition, clinical questions and the concerns of modern medicine concerns have shifted where a role for a new more applied form of CMA would be useful. That applied form means direct presence of medical anthropologists into clinical settings, as well as a patient-centered approach for practicing physicians. In addition, the focus from applied anthropology of the importance of recognizing and working with multiple stakeholders is important in clinical settings (see chapter 6: the leaflet project). The growth of structural approaches is a bridge to reach this objective, which includes finding ways to mediate culture/structure and, from a patient perspective, thinking of illness and suffering. But this perspective takes time and education.

In this book we show not only how the educational models we have developed for premedical undergraduates, medical students, and residents can eventually lead to recognition of cultural and structural issues that underlie patient suffering, but also how applied medical anthropologists can contribute to closing the mismatch gap between physicians and patients, and, hopefully, address the burnout culture in medicine. However, applied anthropologists must integrate some important theoretical contributions of CMA (e.g., Farmer et al. 2006; Krieger et al. 201; Singer 2003) to address limitations in prior efforts of applied medical anthropologists to work in clinical spaces (Chrisman and Maretzki 1982). In this chapter, we propose a new critical, clinically applied anthropology—a Clinically Applied Anthropology 2.0—that integrates CMA concerns for structural violence, as well as concepts from Kleinman et al. (1978) and Hahn (1996) into medical training, patient experience, and approaches to healthcare design and delivery. Medical anthropologists have continued to develop theory and methods that are useful, in novel ways not previously integrated into clinical practice.

More broadly, a clinically applied medical anthropology may also help to resolve tensions between structural and cultural approaches in medical anthropology. There is a continued gap in the culture of biomedical providers, of patients seeking care, and the space created in-between. There are also significant structural determinants and constraints that distribute health and healthcare inequitably across the population. Clinically Applied Anthropology 2.0 attempts to integrate in both models for education and methods to integrate medical anthropologists directly into clinical care spaces.

CMA has sought to separate itself from clinically applied approaches (Chrisman and Maretzki 1982). Each paradigm is assumed to have vastly different underlying assumptions as well as different questions, theoretical grounding, and methodological approaches. However, if clinically applied work is going to offer a new perspective to biomedical systems and providers, integration of aspects of critical theory is useful. On the other hand, if CMA is to remain a relevant and viable perspective, the ability to talk to and work with those outside of the field is important. The application of the concept of structural violence should be extended into our consideration of patient experiences. How does a patient experiencing an illness undergo structural violence when waiting in the ED, when being stigmatized for opioid dependence or for having an illness for which no organic disease can be identified by a provider, or having to utilize a family member or a janitor to attempt language translation, or even to use a professional interpreter each time they need to communicate with healthcare staff? How does this accumulation of non-intentional stressors affect the recovery of an ill patient?

Thus, a new clinically applied medical anthropology might take on healthcare questions that not only need answers at the bedside for patients but also might allow new ways of examining healthcare system failure and provider frustration. A new clinically applied medical anthropology still recognizes the impact and importance of culture but follows Good's suggestions to shift away from emphasizing local "belief systems" (Good 1993). Following the new structuralists and cultural theorists, it instead focuses on the process of how healthcare becomes a stratified commodity with differential outcomes within and across human groups. One focus is on structural violence, structural vulnerability, and how specific phenomenon such as embodiment might help to engage marginalized patient populations, or hidden populations, such as those with previous gunshot wounds who now suffer chronic downstream manifestations (see chapter 11). Clinically applied medical anthropology can also explore ways to improve meaningful healthcare interactions between those that are suffering and those that are providing care by addressing difficult questions surrounding healthcare deservingness (see discussion of these issues around opioid issues in chapter 10).

To revisit critical and clinical medical anthropology approaches, it is also important to revisit the concept of culture—the role of culture in disease and illness, biomedicine as a culture, cultural differences between any patient and any provider (Hahn 1996), as well as the influence of cultural practices versus structural forces in determining access to healthcare, biomedical literacy, and healthcare outcomes. As such, a second important focus is on differing models and expectations between patients and physicians.

The notion of the culture of biomedicine (Hahn 1996) is also important. Latour (1993) suggests that the role of culture is as a complex system in which knowledge is produced and viewed (the physician-patient encounter reproduces the EM culture each time, 30 encounters a shift). As humans become more interconnected, our attention can turn to a biocultural/biopolitical synthesis that instead addresses how humans not only explain the world around them and organize naturally occurring diseases and behaviors, but also produce and reproduce systems of power that generates more risk to human health than any biophysiological disease model. This is an extremely important concept in modern healthcare. Physicians know what to do for a stroke and myocardial infarction, but what to do with the health situations that have no ICD-10 code, no core measure, no best practice, or a just-evolving evidence-based medicine? Are those patients' issues less valid or less deserving? Their biology less real? If a physician culture exists and opioid user culture exists, can a new structure be built collaboratively (following Kleinman et al.'s now 40-year-old suggestions [1978]) between healthcare workers and medical anthropologists that defines a new, coproduced, object and locus for treatment?

Human culture is responsible for the creation of political economies that marginalize groups of humans. Where we find that marginalization, we find local cultural variation to account for these stratified differences. In addition, marginalized groups are where the next risk factor for human disease or well-known epidemiological killer will emerge, as the marginalized are often the first to die in large numbers of disease (e.g., people who inject drugs and homosexual men in the AIDs epidemic in the United States in the 1980s). Marginalized groups are also the last to have full access to preventive measures, education, and behaviors that lead to shifts and improvements in poor outcomes for endemic chronic disease states (such as coronary artery disease and diabetes) (Farmer 2003). Human culture—with a big C perhaps?—through the classic definition of shared patterns of behavior and socially transmitted learning allows endless reproduction of power structures. These structures provide a bio-loop to culture and to human biology, reinforcing structural power and structural violence, but also directly affecting inheritable genetic changes among people faced with physiological stress and poor health, even creating observable changes in local biologies (Gravlee 2009).

Culture has the potential to allow imagined structures and structural bridges that close the social distance (Madaras 2019) between groups (anthropologists and physicians, physicians, and patients)—a distance created partially through preexisting structures of the cultural artifacts of ICD-10 codes (specific billing codes that define a patient encounter), core measures (compliance metrics regulated by third-party payers and the federal government for payment), and the medical curriculum. An imagined future might shed light on hidden populations in medical clinics as anthropologists and physicians work together to create pathways for opioid care, sickle cell disease management, HCV, injection drug use, mental health, and downstream sequelae of patients with prior gunshot wounds. While the biology might be "real" and "out there" to be discovered, what biology we acknowledge shifts over time.

Colin Hemmings has pointed out that "medical anthropology has helped articulate the problems of medicine but not provided realistic solutions" (Hemmings 2010). The goal of medical anthropology should not only be to improve the biomedical system but also to advance the explanation of sociocultural variation in medicine. Theory must also be developed and that theory that has been developed, without the goal of specific healthcare improvements, can now be useful to applied anthropologists working with healthcare providers. For example, Heather Henderson's work reviewed in chapter 10 describes how the "learned helplessness" of patients with opioid use disorder is perpetuated by the same feelings among the law enforcement officers, physicians, and healthcare systems that encounter those patients. She demonstrates how that learned helplessness reproduces stigma surrounding substance use (Henderson 2018). In that chapter, we outline how this ethnographically obtained knowledge was used, along with how syndemic concepts were advanced to colocate treatment strategies and to also propose new ways to view entanglements inherent to the distribution of patients in the ED. Similar to the research and development section of a manufacturing company or biotech, there must also be some application of this theory to practice, or what is the point? But another issue is if working in a clinical setting means that the anthropologist has become subservient to a physician (as implied by Scheper-Hughes 1990)? The premise of this question assumes ownership of the clinical space by the physician. However, the triple aim approach takes away that ownership in reference to the patient experience, opening the door wide for collaboration in healthcare settings within an interdisciplinary team, which must include clinically applied anthropologists.

There are two assumptions to moving forward with a clinical/critical synthesis and a new clinically applied medical anthropology. First, as a white male physician-anthropologist (JWW), I am an insider and part of the biomedical culture described here. In addition, I would suggest that most medical anthropologists working in the United States are also encultured into that model, at least as patients or potential patients, and, if working on research questions in the field, also as workers within the overarching biomedical empire. Thus, we move past the question of whether our work reproduces a biomedical model. In a sense, yes, it does. However, considering the work of Good (1992), we argue that one can study within this frame while also being able to critique it. Also, if we can use this same lens of analysis on other health knowledge systems or para-biomedical systems (e.g., homeopathy, witchcraft, Ayurveda, integrative medicine), then this same approach can be applied to biomedicine (Good 1992).

The second assumption implicit here, and which differs from some critical approaches, is that we are not concerned with whether we are medicalizing research questions or observed phenomenon. Yes, we are. As a matter of fact, for many of us, the interest in biomedicine viewed from an anthropological perspective is not that we feel that biomedicine does not have the potential for alleviating human suffering. But instead, we want tools and theory that ground us in a critique of how biomedicine falls short in improving the lives of many potential beneficiaries. Thus, while Scheper-Hughes (1990) worries about how we as medical anthropologists are viewed (pawns? Cogs in the wheel? of biomedicine), we are instead concerned with whether all patients have equitable access to the potential healing properties of our medical system, that our medical system moves in directions that ultimately leads to more inclusion across cultural and structural boundaries, and that providers and patients meet each other in a space (mediated by the medical anthropologist) that may open new ways of healing.

"How does this help me?" "What are we supposed to do with this?" "This is not my job!" Those are all common responses received when talking with physicians about ways to integrate cultural and structural competence into clinical encounters. Applied anthropologists, if we are going to talk with others outside of the discipline, now have a responsibility to answer these questions, whether that be in the macro clinical setting (healthcare systems and the development of the clinical gaze), or in the context of individual encounters between physicians and patients. We help healthcare providers include structural and cultural approaches to understanding human disease, emphasizing the role of structure in predicting healthcare outcomes and disease stratification, while emphasizing the role culture has for making meaning, embodiment, and suffering. Both structure and culture are ultimately critical in effecting patient compliance with physician recommendations.

This may take time. Both of us have been co-teaching a patient-physician interaction course for five years to premedical students (chapter 3). Many of those students are now in medical school. The course focuses on developing a patient-centered lens early in training with a recognition of how structure predicts patient encounters and how culture interacts to produce meaning within those encounters. In addition, we have both also begun working with internal medicine residents and conducting patient shadowing workshops. The goal is that, over time, the clinical gaze will begin to shift, so that questions of medical anthropological applicability become obvious to the provider, as we anthropologists continue to offer valuable applied insight into system-based and patient-level clinical encounters. As such, our goals bridge older and newer approaches to medical anthropology; we seek to observe and critique—but also to disrupt and change healthcare in patient-centered radical ways.

Chapter 3

Working with Undergraduate Premedical and Anthropology Graduate Students

The logic for considering patients and physicians as two different cultures is well established (Kleinman et al. 1978; Hahn 1996). The challenge, then, becomes how to bridge this gap and establish an effective means of cross-cultural communication. While Kleinman et al. (1978) suggest an understanding of each other's explanatory models, we feel that a more in-depth approach is appropriate. Our informal conversations with physicians indicate that those who have experienced a serious health issue of their own or within their immediate families have a better understanding of the patient's perspective and of illness. However, many medical students and residents (physicians in training) are young and have not experienced much interaction with the healthcare system outside of visiting their pediatrician, student health clinic, and, perhaps, primary care physician in preparation for college or medical school. Dempsey (2017), an executive at Press-Ganey, also noted this pattern but uses the term "suffering" instead of illness. The use of the words "suffering" and "illness" is important to link as many current authors have used the term "suffering" often to capture similar, but perhaps broader, understanding of the dichotomy between disease and illness outlined by Kleinman et al. in the late 1970s.

Understanding that suffering and illness perspectives are linked helps further solidify a bridge between earlier concepts of clinically applied anthropology and more recent paradigm shifts toward critically applied anthropology. The physician focuses on biological disease through a lens of training in line with biomedicine while the patient suffers because of a gap in explanatory models between disease and illness/suffering, and a mismatch in encounter expectations. Further, there is the structural violence of biopower that places the patient within a bureaucratic system of hallway beds, language interpretation variability, and differential access. In addition, the structural determinants of health explain many differences in health outcomes (e.g., housing status, poverty, mental health, and psychological trauma) and all make up the everyday structural violence of patient suffering, embodied in their illness presentation.

Patients are frustrated by a mismatch of expectations during the clinical encounter. They continue to feel a deficit in addressing illness and complain of impersonal treatment and lack of attention to their concerns. For their part, physicians are frustrated by nonmedical healthcare issues (e.g., social determinants) and institution and third-party reimbursement demands to improve the patient experience, while meeting a number of compliance benchmarks. Additionally, physicians are rushed and feel their work has lost its meaning, emphasizing a mismatch in training and clinical reality. Within the context of value-based purchasing as part of the triple aim in healthcare to improve quality of care while controlling cost, patient satisfaction scores have become an important part of both institution level and provider level concern given implications for reimbursement (Wilson et al. 2019).

The challenge then becomes one of imbuing such understandings in providers, without waiting for them to have a similar personal situation of a serious health issue themselves or in a close family member.

Approaching this problem from an applied anthropological perspective, the challenge can be reframed as one of how to enable one group to understand the culture of another, a classic applied anthropological concern. Our answer and approach are also based in the basics of anthropology—participant observation. Participant observation helps the outsider understand another culture by participating in it, but remaining a partial outsider, who can analyze and reflect upon their experiences. It is this perspective and method we used in designing the 15-week, undergraduate class, "Research Experience in Patient Provide Interaction."

We felt that anthropological approaches could address multiple problems related to current training of physicians. Premed students have numerous requirements and little time to take medical anthropology courses. They are also expected to be involved in research and to shadow physicians. Admission to medical school has also become much more competitive.

Our goal was to integrate medical anthropological theory and methods into training of future physicians so that a patient experience approach will be hardwired into their training, preventing later mismatch/potential burnout from frustration in meeting patient expectations. Participants learn medical anthropology, but the key part of the project involves what we have termed "patient shadowing," which parallels the standard medical training activity of physician shadowing. However, we structure "patient shadowing" to be anthropological participant observation and reflection. Thus, the anthropological difference is our use of medical anthropological theory and participant observation that enables the understanding of the patient's perspective (Wilson et al. 2019).

The class began through the desire of both authors to change the way physicians were trained. The project is ongoing and has developed several parts beginning in 2016. We first developed a course for premedical honors students and then created two follow-up courses for students who have taken the first course and wish to continue to work with us (this chapter). More recently, we also developed a two-day workshop for internal medicine residents at the University of South Florida (USF) and, in 2019, developed a longitudinal voluntary experience for medical students at the USF Morsani Medical School curriculum (chapter 5). The medical student experience emphasizes patient shadowing during the first year of medical school as part of an elective experience that students choose from several options. The offering was requested by medical school first-year course leaders after our own student alumni began entering medical school and talking about the great experience of patient shadowing and how powerful that impact was on their early thinking and training during their education.

The Physician-Patient Interaction course for premed USF Honors College students exposes participants to medical anthropological readings and then requires students to do participant observation in the Tampa General Hospital (TGH) Emergency Department (ED). The ED was chosen given the access provided to the site through JWW, a practicing Emergency Medicine (EM) physician and administrator in the department, as well as the likelihood that students would encounter a broad range of issues pertaining to disease, illness, and suffering in that fieldwork.

The specific topics addressed in the course include an introduction to EM, followed by readings related to a qualitative research and a Quality Improvement (QI) project in which the students participate. During the course, specific didactics also focus on human subject research, IRB, QI, and the challenges of Health Insurance Portability and Accountability Act (HIPAA). During the semester, students complete a simulated IRB proposal. In addition, all students complete human subject research certification (CITI Website) and are added to an active firearm research protocol approved by a local IRB (USF IRB Pro0003945). Research ethics are also covered prior to the students along with basic concepts in research design. After an introduction and overview of these research concepts, students learn more about participant observation as well as techniques for writing field notes.

Other topics covered in the course include a background in the importance of the patient experience and the patient perspective in healthcare, as well as key concepts in medical anthropology (illness versus disease, the notion of differing physician and patient perspectives, the biocultural perspective in illness causation, worldview and value orientation, biomedicine as a culture, and ethnomedicine). We still assign the 1978 article by Arthur Kleinman et al. that outlines mismatches in explanatory models of disease and illness as well as the basic issues challenging healthcare (expense, unsatisfied patients). When students read this article, we ask, what did you notice? Most point out that the article is over 40 years old. The students (especially the medical residents who see patients every day) then point out and agree that nothing has changed, or things may have gotten worse in healthcare since publication of this article. In other words, approaching problems in healthcare the same way we always have is not working. Our belief is that these interdisciplinary approaches bring a patient-centered approach to problem-solving, and hard-wire that into the next generation of physicians. They also simultaneously address contemporary problems in healthcare that are not just of theoretical concern to the social scientist but of actual praxes concern to the physician and medical system.

Literature on social determinants of health and the importance of culture and an anthropological approach to patient suffering is also considered through readings and discussion. The final classes are devoted to hands-on analysis of the data collected (laptops are brought to class; faculty as well as graduate students are present to assist in coding and statistical analysis). The students then prepare a report documenting the experiences and findings from that semester and, for the projects that span a semester, situate their findings in the larger context of previous classes. The students do an oral presentation, and we later compile a formal written report of their findings. The oral presentation is done for hospital administration, ED leadership and leadership from the USF Honors College, including the dean who has supported creation, implementation, and continuation of the course based on our ability to place students directly into a community real-world learning experience and prepare them for medical school simultaneously.

The course includes two projects, a longitudinal QI project which focused on patients who leave the ED without being seen by a physician. There have been multiple iterations and different topics for the research project) over the years. In year 1 (Spring 2016), students completed qualitative, open-ended interviews with patients in the waiting room about patient concerns during the visit. The results of that work developed into the leaflet project in year 2 (see chapter 6) which focused on using patient-generated data to create patient-centered information. Beginning in Fall 2018, we have had students participate in an ongoing research project involving firearm injuries (see chapter 11 for more detail on the results of this project). Admittedly, there was some trepidation in having students engage patients, physicians, and staff with more acute injury or history of significant trauma. However, our experiences with our students in the first few years of the course allowed trust to be established between ED staff and the authors that students could perform well in the ED/healthcare environment. Patient narratives regarding their own personal encounters with firearm violence, and the emotions those narratives can generate for the patients recounting their stories and answering questions, are also not without some specific concerns. We teach students in the late teens or early 20s. Many have never heard stories of such incredible tragedy and suffering. In addition, the ED itself is an environment of "bare life" (Agamben 1999). Many of our students see death for the first time. Sometimes in the ED, death is not even the most tragic as students also witness domestic violence, sex trafficking, arrest and separation, and acute mental health crisis, bringing to light places in the world many of the students did not know still existed or existed in their own backyard. The reflections of the GSW interviews by the students, as well as the discussions around everyday events in the ED, have led us to formalize debriefings into the course throughout the semester.

For the GSW research project, each student interviews two ED patients who have gunshot wounds using an interview guide originally designed by the class. The GSW patient interview takes place either in the ED or the hospital floor. All interviews are done in pairs, so each student gets to sit in on four interviews. Each student submits field notes (detailed observations) on these interviews.

The emphasis of the GSW study is on the downstream sequalae following GSW injuries including the social cost of being shot, as well as the respondents' views on their treatment and firearm policy before and after the injury. Our goal is that this specific patient-generated data will lead us to propose patient-informed intervention hypotheses in the future that can also be tested using mixed methods approach. We believe that this cycle of patient-informed data gathering, hypothesized intervention using the patient-informed data, and then test of that intervention using further mixed methods approaching involving patients are the keys to new ways of improving patient experience. The sickle cell disease project (chapter 8), leaflet project (chapter 6), and opioid project (chapter 10) in this monograph are all examples of this methodology.

The longitudinal QI approach offers a way to ensure students access to the ED to conduct participant observation while attempting to help the hospital find ways to improve the quality of care. The nature of long-term, continuous observation and data collection in QI lends itself well to our undergraduate semester model. This also enables us to ensure that access remains in place each year that we teach the course without having to restart all the administrative requirements to do an investigation in the hospital or clinical space.

Our QI aspect of the work utilizes students conducting participating observation in waiting room, triage, and other ED clinical spaces to gather information about why patients would consider leaving the ED without being seen to inform future interventions targeted at decreasing LWBS%. This specific QI lends itself well to the methods of participant observation and opens spaces that would be otherwise difficult to access for an investigator secondary to HIPAA (e.g., the waiting room). Patients who leave prior to being seen are known to often return to the ED sicker than on the previous encounter. Every patient who leaves the ED prior to evaluation also represents lost revenue for the institution and providers. A federal law, the Emergency Medicine Treatment and Labor Act mandates a medical screening exam (MSE) by a qualified medical provider for all people that enter an ED (or come within hundreds of feet seeking care). If a patient leaves before the MSE is initiated (by a physician or other provider), that patient is considered to have left without being seen (LWBS). The number of patients who leave without being seen is tracked as a throughput metric (LWBS%) and reported to the Centers for Medicare and Medicaid Services (CMS) and available as public data (CMS Hospital Compare Site).

For the QI project, students are each assigned two blocks of participant observation. One participant observation block (three hours) is with an assigned physician in a physician-shadowing capacity. Upon arriving in the ED, the students ask for this physician and report to the pod (area of the ED) where that physician is working clinically. The other block is based in the ED waiting room. Students spend one hour at the security desk watching arrival and processing, one hour at the pivot desk, and one hour in the waiting room, observing and talking informally with patients (especially those they've "met" at the pivot desk). Each participant observation block is three hours (six hours total).

Students are also assigned to follow two patients through their visit. The patient shadowing takes place during assigned four-hour shifts with a specific physician. They go to the pod where the assigned physician is working. During a clinic shift with the physician, the student interviews a patient that is assigned to them by that physician. The requirement for this new patient is to be one that has only gone through the triage process but has not yet been seen by the treating clinical team. The student follows the patient everywhere and to everything (diagnostic studies including imaging such as CT scans, X-ray, and ultrasonography). This shadowing process takes approximately four hours for each patient encounter. In QI and healthcare system metrics, this time is the "room to disposition time." In other words, this is the period of time during the patient's ED encounter in which they are placed into a treatment space to see a physician (e.g., a room); are seen by the treating physician; undergo a history and physical exam by the treating physician; have orders placed for labs and other diagnostic studies; undergo procedures (e.g., sutures for laceration repair, lumbar puncture to evaluate for meningitis); have consultant services see, examine, or conduct specialized exams or procedures; receive medications and other supportive care for the underlying condition (e.g., IV fluids); and ultimately found to need further hospitalization or can be discharged back home (or back to a skilled nursing facility or other institution). On average, this room to disposition time is approximately three to four hours of the overall ED encounter.

After each session of participation observation/shadowing, the student writes and turns in field notes on their experiences. In class, later, the students also discuss their experiences, debrief, and then interview the physician who treated that patient. The physician interviews take place during a physician panel near the end of the semester. Physicians that spent time with the students in the course attend one of the class sessions to answer questions that arose during the patient encounter or clinical shift or questions that arose as the student reflected on field notes and readings for the course.

The student also asks each patient two formal questions toward the end of their time with them: Now you've been here a while and so have I! Sometimes people leave the ED without seeing a doctor—is that something you would think of doing? Why or why not?

We recognize that there are limitations to this approach as a study designed to analyze reasons for leaving without being seen (given that these patients did not leave and, as far as the student knows, not been planning to leave). However, the approach does allow data collection that builds a rich distribution of possible reasons for that patient would consider leaving without being seen in the future or may have done so in the past. We believe this type of data collection during a clinical encounter provides data that can inform future hypothesized interventions to reduce LWBS%. In addition, our focus on improving the quality of care at the institution allows a less restrictive environment for participant observation to take place within the HIPAA (HIPAA leading to increased privacy concerns within hospital spaces). This project also allows students to meet premedical application requirements (shadowing, research, patient contact) while also integrating a patient focused lens early in their training. Without exception, the students report that this is the most meaningful and impactful part of the course.

We developed the QI project focusing on the ED LWBS rate for the fall 2019 class as a way of formalizing the participant observation exercises that had always been a part of the class. In doing this we had several concerns, the major one being that we did not want to overfocus the students and give them a formal questionnaire or set of topics to observe (maintaining the empiric nature of anthropological research). For this reason, students were only given two questions to ask and only at the end of their patient observations. In addition, by making this a formal QI project, we achieved two important goals. The first was that we now had a clearly defined focus and product to offer the hospital—and on a topic of great concern to them given the safety and revenue implications when patients leave prior to a MSE being completed. The second was that as a QI project, we gained the freedom to present the data from the participant observation, something that our IRB would not approve for a research project (see chapter 4 for more discussion of IRB issues). The project thus worked much better than it ever had before and focused the students on a way that was helpful, but not restrictive or antithetical to anthropological methods.

Admission into the course is competitive (even though we did not anticipate this). When we first offered the course, we sent out an email to the advisers in the USF Honors College and Department of Anthropology alerting premedical students that the course would be offered. We hoped to get 10 to 12 people interested in the course but instead received 100 emails back from students wanting to take the course. This forced us to create an ad-hoc application review process that we have now formalized into a course application that we use each year to select students. The competitiveness of the course has ensured that we are able to select students who are likely to go to medical school (since the goal of this course is to hardwire a patient-centered approach early in training of physicians). This includes a competitive GPA and relevant course work, in combination with a background of taking at least one anthropology or social science course, demonstrating some openness to approaches outside of "hard" sciences. In addition, given the requirements for the course, we often focus on selecting upper-level students, usually juniors who have had time to complete some of the background prerequisites, but who also still have time to potentially continue with us in the honors thesis course taught each year after ED-based course. We also admit a small number of medical anthropology graduate students into the class, helping them to develop an interest in hospital-based projects with a patient-centered focus and, potentially, setting those students up for applied careers in the patient experience or patient relations departments of U.S. hospitals (an underrecognized venue for applied medical anthropologists).

The course has now been taught multiple times and many of our prior students have matriculated into medical school. We consent those students to remain part of an ongoing longitudinal cohort study that considers the downstream term impacts of the patient-centered approach on clinical training—an attempt to shift the clinical gaze over time.

Review of course evaluations reveals that the entire semester-long course is a valuable experience for the students; however, patient shadowing is the most cited specific aspect of the course that provides a life-changing experience and memorable encounter. As one student explained,

> I was unsure about doing the patient observations. However, as we started reading more about problems in the healthcare system and the ED, I started

> realizing the importance of the patient perspective. Once I started realizing how important it was to consider the patient perspective, I became more open to the idea of doing the waiting room observations. However, being open to the idea of doing patient observations did not mean I was completely ready to do it. . . . When it was time to go to the ED, I gave myself a pep-talk that got me onto the second floor of [the hospital] and walking towards the ED, but it only lasted long enough for me to find the nearest restroom and run inside and have a minor panic attack. After the second pep-talk, I managed to complete the assignment, but I was still worried about how I was going to do the assignment the following week. Nevertheless, I persisted, mostly because I know I was going to be graded and I had no other choice. And honestly the experience I had doing the patient and physician shadowing was unparalleled . . . I left . . . with a new understanding of what it felt like to be alone during one of the most vulnerable periods of someone's life. I also left . . . with a new sense of how to be a better health care provider.

In a required reflection paper at the end of the course, we ask the students to identify what aspects of the course they feel will be most important to them as physicians. A thematic analysis of the responses of four classes (N = 68) indicates that 82% noted the importance of the patient experience, 34% discussed the distinction between illness and disease, 32% noted the differences between patient and physician perspectives, and 56% discussed the importance of anthropology, culture, and other social determinants of health.

The semester-long patient-physician interaction course is followed by an optional class called Designing Research for Health and Clinical Studies. The second course is only open to students who have taken the first class with us and is designed for students who want to do health or clinically related research for their honors thesis.

During the Designing Research for Health and Clinical Studies course, students can create and complete an honors thesis project on a health/clinical-related topic, with access to a clinical site, hospital patients, and medical records, if appropriate.

The course arose after JWW and RDB were both accepting honors students who were at different phases of their research, requiring the two faculty members to repeat didactic material, remain in a constant state of hospital credentialing, and lose the opportunity for students to be involved in peer review, critical analysis, and group learning when designing research questions and proposals. Our research design course focuses on utilizing mixed methods to address healthcare problems in a way that is different from strictly clinical and quantitative or public health/population based/secondary data analysis level approaches. Instead, students develop mostly prospective or observational studies that involve both quantitative data collection and analysis but also which utilize participant observation, interviewing, thematic coding, and other qualitative approaches to research questions and hypotheses. In addition, publicly available data is explored during class sessions to teach research methods and to explore investigator choices in research design to help students develop an honors prospectus.

The course begins with the students usually having no clear idea of what they want to work on or do for an honors thesis, other than knowing they want to do something related to healthcare and are willing to utilize the mixed methods approaches introduced by JWW and RDB in the first course. Over the course of the semester, the students' research questions become clear and precise and, when appropriate, are formalized into a hypothesis with clear predictions that guide the development of methods and ideas for how to test their hypothesis or answer the research question. Each week students re-share their research topic and other students, as well as faculty (JWW and RDB), ask questions and provide feedback in a supportive critical format.

The class covers principles of research design; topics include key elements of a research proposal, health service/quality, cross-sectional, case control, clinical research and retrospective research, IRB and ethnics issues, randomized control trials, approaches to data analysis, and race as a unit of analysis. Each faculty member also discusses their own successful and unsuccessful past grant and research proposals and share personal experiences from years of research work. The goal of the course is for the student to finalize a research question and develop that question into a formal thesis prospectus following our university IRB format.

But particularly for undergraduate student thesis projects, an issue has been the length of time necessary to get a project through the many levels of approval at the hospital and through IRB review. Initially, our goal was for students to move a project from idea to prospectus during the first part of the semester and then submit the study to IRB at the end of the semester (as the final capstone) with IRB approval the next semester allowing the student to begin conducting research at that time. However, the turnaround time for these projects often took the entire next semester. In addition, having the student listed as PI was not ideal for several reasons. First, the student as PI is not a known researcher to IRB, with no formed relationships or history of trust developed with that staff or the hospital. This may create a higher standard or increased level of scrutiny since a student may not fully understand the importance of human subject's protection or the need to not commit protocol deviations (or the regulatory steps necessary in the event of a protocol deviation). Second, students simply have many competing obligations and shifting emphasis on what and when something is important leading to delays in turnaround of requested IRB or hospital documents. Finally, as researchers with a serious interest in helping solve ongoing problems in medicine, a model of student projects with that student as PI was not very impactful.

Another issue is that upon submission to the IRB, honors thesis projects also require approval from the hospital to ensure that the research is compliant (has IRB approval, student is credentialed, no significant disruption on clinical operations, no significant need for funding or supplies that has not been addressed in the protocol). After IRB protocol or protocol-amendment approval, hospital approval, credentialing (including both hospital credentialing involving HIPAA training and orientation to universal precautions and infection control), students can finally begin to collect new data in the ED or other associated hospital space.

As a result of these time-consuming issues, we have moved to a set of longitudinal projects in which the faculty (JWW and RDB) are the PIs. This allows the faculty to develop long-term projects that can be completed over multiple semesters, not just one, adding data in a serial manner as a student joins the project. Each semester, the student who joins an ongoing project can create an addendum to an already approved IRB protocol that carves out space of interest and intellectual property for that student. For example, if we want to examine cultural and structural variation in hemoglobin A1C control in diabetics, one student might spend time asking about time spent exercising in good and poorly controlled diabetics, while another might compare a group of Southeast Asian patients to a group of African American patients. Each student though will maintain some shared interview questions and collect a core set of similar data, adding to a growing data set over time. However, an IRB amendment allows that student to add some specific data collection elements (e.g., number of hours spent exercising per week). That student can write about the overall project and then analyze the data they collected, framing the analysis within their own question, but also considering all the data for context. RDB and JWW are then able to grow the data set and consider broader patterns and help guide future students in directions that might address gaps in the longitudinal work.

Undergraduate projects to date include the following:

- Ahan Kayastha, Sonal Sian: Investigation of the Differences in Lifestyle and Self-Care Practices Among Good vs. Poor Glycemic Control Non-Hispanic Black Diabetic Patients
- Maya Subramanian, Sheon Baby: Coronary Heart Disease and the Female Patient Experience—A Qualitative Approach
- Keertana Nimmagadda, Victoria Sands: Emergency Medical Service Naloxone Preparedness
- Kirtan Patel, Shalini Jose: Investigating Physician-Patient Interactions Based on the Presence or Absence of Family During Consultations in the Emergency Department

- Kimberly Van: Barriers to Diet Adherence in Newly Diagnosed Type 2 Diabetic Patients: The Patient and Educator Perspective
- Meera Navadia: A Mixed Methods Analysis of a Quality Improvement Program at Tampa General Hospital Designed to Reduce Utilization in a Group of Multi-visit Patients: Can Patients Experience Data Improve Care Coordination?
- Lucy Garner: The Analysis of Patient-Physician Interaction at Tampa General Hospital
- Mery Yanez: The Perception Paradox: Experiences of Spanish-Speaking Patients in the Emergency Department
- Danielle Melton: A Look at Patient Preference for Emergency Medical Care

We have also had two anthropology graduate students do MA theses in the clinical setting of the TGH ED:

- Heather Henderson: "I Am More than My Addiction": Perceptions of Stigma and Access to Care in Acute Opioid Crisis. MA Thesis. Department of Anthropology. USF. Tampa, Florida, 2018.
- Seichi Villalona: Looking Beyond Patient Satisfaction: Experiences of Spanish-Speaking Patients Seeking Non-Urgent Care in an Emergency Department. MA Thesis. Department of Anthropology. University of South Florida. Tampa, Florida, 2019

While we have read about other courses for premedical students, such as that at Cornell (Goldstein et al. 2014), which focuses on opportunities for undergraduates to shadow physicians in different specialties, we are unaware of any courses like ours which incorporate physician and patient shadowing, as well as research/QI projects in the context of a course for premed students. Nor are we aware of courses which prepare undergraduates for clinically based research. We hope our models will encourage others to consider such activities.

Chapter 4

Challenges of Clinically Applied Anthropology Education and Research

Contributions by Emily Holbrook

Over the last six years, we created two courses and integrated both premedical undergraduate students and graduate students directly into a clinical space while also expanding our work to emphasize patient experience-based approaches for medical students early in their clinical training and medical residents in their second year of postgraduate training. The physical placement of premedical students into patient rooms and anthropology graduate students directly into hospital clinical areas matches our theoretical interest to shift the clinical gaze toward patient focus by initiating understanding of suffering and patient experience early in medical education while also demonstrating a previously less emphasized or considered role of the medical anthropologist not as a para-clinical observer only, but as an applied acting member of future healthcare teams (Wilson et al. 2019).

The significant federal laws around patient privacy and security create hospital entry burdens for nonclinical faculty, much less premedical student who are 20 year olds. However, our partnership and persistence has allowed these students, semester after semester, to work and learn within a clinical space. That clinical space is also not just any space—we have successfully worked with students around patients in a busy urban Emergency Department (ED) and Level 1 trauma center where daily patient volume is high, and encounters are often highly charged and acute. We have been able to move students through multiple areas of that clinical space as a group, as individuals, as observers, and as autonomous investigators working to answer important research questions both at the undergraduate and graduate level. This has been challenging to initiate, implement, and then grow. However, even with several significant challenges, we have essentially been successful and now have expanded into other areas of the hospital and into the outpatient clinic system. We have been able to do this by creating a team that includes multiple institutions, organizations, and individuals (JW, RB, graduate assistant support, research assistants (RAs) who work in the ED, hospital administrative support, university support). We owe a tremendous amount of gratitude to Emily Holbrook (an anthropology PhD candidate at time of this writing and our graduate student assistant) who, each year, has continued to solidify her relationships across the university, hospital, and physician practice management group, as well as the local University of South Florida (USF) IRB. Without Emily, we would have had difficulty streamlining and organizing a credentialing and access approach for students. Emily also became an expert at the regulatory requirements around local IRB, especially navigating investigator-initiated interdisciplinary studies that do not fit well in the traditional binary of medical or social science IRB review assignment. Emily has contributed significantly to writing this chapter. Other departments, divisions, and organizations that have had significant involvement in course success are the USF Department of Anthropology, TEAMHealth (the physician practice group), the USF Honors College, the USF Morsani College of Medicine, and the USF Emergency Medicine (EM) residency program, as well as the USF Internal Medicine program.

THE TEAM

This is the most complex part of a complex project. Team teaching is always a challenge, and in this case, the two individuals who are involved in this project are perfectly situated to make this project a success. Baer has over 30 years of teaching and research experience in medical anthropology. Wilson has an MA in anthropology and is a practicing emergency physician and administrator (medical director) with his medical doctorate (MD). So, both faculty leaders have a foot in each other's universe. In addition, between Wilson and the Anthropology Department, we have always had one graduate assistant assigned to the class (we discuss the activities of this assistant in working on credentialing and permissions for the research/Quality Improvement (QI) activities below). The graduate assistant also creates an online shared calendar (we use Google) for the class to schedule activities at Tampa General Hospital (TGH) (patient shadowing, physician assignments, interviewing, etc.). Wilson is also the research director in the ED and operates a clinical trials program that generates revenue that is used to pay RAs who have routine duties that involve screening ED patients for ongoing trials but also support our course projects. Many of these RAs are former course students that have graduated but are in a transition time ("gap year") between college and medical school. The RAs monitor patients arriving at the ED and notify the class of those who fit our research/QI sample criteria (e.g., patients with gunshot wound injuries or those with prior gunshot wound injuries presenting to the ED with other complaints). This is often done utilizing the GroupMe application (GroupMe 2011) with a shared group among the RAs and students in our class that semester.

UNIVERSITY SUPPORT

This has been critical. The chair of the Anthropology Department has permitted Baer to teach the classes as part of her normal assignment, reasoning that the classes tightly tie anthropology to the STEM focus of the university. The course is cross-listed with Honors courses, and the dean of the Honor's College provides a stipend for Wilson, as he does not have a teaching assignment at USF and, given the complexities of EM culture and contracting, not able to simply reduce some percentage of his assigned FTE duties at the hospital. Eric Eisenberg, the dean of the College of Arts and Sciences (in which the Department of Anthropology is housed) has also been integral in support and growth of the course. Eisenberg specializes in communication, and his prior research has mostly been done in the ED and focused on narratives, storytelling, and meaning-making in triage and during the patient visit (Roscoe, Eisenberg, and Forde 2016). In the past, Wilson facilitated and supported the use of the ED as a field site for a PhD student (Forde) working with Eisenberg on similar communication issues. Each year, Eisenberg comes and presents his work with the student. The presence of Eisenberg, Wilson, and Baer evolves into a panel discussion about healthcare, and is usually cited as the favorite class meeting by the students given the three experienced and different perspectives on modern challenges in healthcare.

HOSPITAL ADMINISTRATIVE SUPPORT

Jason Wilson is the director of Research within the Department of Internal Medicine, Division of EM—a role that has obligations for an academic EM residency program and to the hospital. In addition, the ED Division chief and medical director also lectures in the class on his experience as a provider in cross-cultural medical settings (New Zealand), and has been supportive of the ED projects. EDs have multiple administrative and leadership positions and nursing is an important stakeholder both in access to the site as well as to the types of questions we ask and the data we collect. The nursing director is the hospital side director of the department, and her support has been invaluable to allowing this course to take place and work within the ED.

Hospital leadership has also been interested and supportive in our project as administrators ranging from the chief medical officer, chief quality officer, chief operating officer, and director of Patient Experience have all attended our presentations and contributed valuable insight to the course—especially staff from the patient experience office.

As part of the course, staff in patient experience and patient relations have been asked to speak to the students regarding their work in TGH and the importance of the patient-physician interaction. Patient relations and patient experience staff also regularly attend the year-end presentation and engage with the students about their results and analyses.

IRB, HOSPITAL COMPLIANCE, AND STUDENT CREDENTIALING

This has been the most challenging part of our projects. Students must be credentialed as researchers to observe in the ED. However, given the ever-evolving environment of hospital medicine, Health Insurance Portability and Accountability Act (HIPAA), and legal corporate compliance regulatory shifts, this process is continually changing, and we frequently find ourselves using outdated forms that have been updated and changed without our knowledge. Often, we have been asked for new information partway through the credentialing process. Along with changes to the forms, to whom we submit the paperwork has also changed, frequently without our knowledge. To be credentialed, each student completes a packet of paperwork that needs to be signed by Wilson. They also submit a signed and dated CV/resume and a badge request form. Students are also required to complete human subjects research training utilizing the Collaborative Institutional Training Initiative online course offered through a subscription maintained by the university. However, the required courses (basic human subjects research and/or Good Clinical Practice) have also shifted between student cohorts and types of students (i.e., honors thesis or graduate students with investigator-initiated projects are required to do more training).

After the initial paperwork has been approved by the hospital, students complete a set of online training courses that cover universal precautions, HIPAA, and other important elements of safety and corporate compliance. Transcripts from those courses are then submitted to the Office of Clinical Research (OCR) and Human Resources department at the hospital. Personnel, course requirements, and mandatory information/applications have changed more than once over the years of teaching this course. While the changes do not necessarily complicate the credentialing process from the students' perspective, it does make the process harder for the team. We often update our instructions to students with little notice and have, on occasion, relayed outdated information that we had to later correct.

For research projects conducted as part of the classes, both IRB and TGH review are required. However, we often find one group objecting to what the other is requiring, and/or questioning what the other has already approved. However, since initiating the course, the hospital and the university research offices have more formally merged, helping to streamline some of these administrative burdens.

Our greatest challenge has been to enable students to do participant observation in the ED waiting room and in patient rooms—two activities we feel are necessary to solid applied clinical medical anthropology and training of patient-centered physicians. Approval for this activity has been more problematic than approval for the administration of questionnaires or open-ended interviews. The main issue of concern comes down to student exposure to private health information. HIPAA of 1996 led to enhanced protection of personal health information (PHI). For research purposes, PHI is usually considered to be any identifying feature of a patient and has been summarized as 18 key elements including names, dates (except year), telephone numbers, geographic data (units below state level including zip codes and address), fax numbers, social security numbers, email addresses, medical record numbers, account numbers, health plan beneficiary numbers, certificate/license numbers, license plates or other vehicle identifiers/serial numbers, web URLs, device identifiers/serial numbers, internet protocol addresses, full face photos/comparable images, biometric data (retinal scan, fingerprints), any unique identifying number or code (Loyola, 18 HIPAA Identifiers). Our local IRB has determined that HIPAA protects patients in the waiting room and in patient rooms to a higher degree than patients would be protected as people outside of the hospital. In other words, by entering a hospital environment, patients (and indeed any person, such as a family member accompanying the patient) have higher expectations for privacy that are protected by HIPAA. It should be emphasized that all our students undergo hospital required HIPAA training through a series of online, interactive modules. In addition, required paperwork also includes a patient privacy agreement in which students agree to any legal consequences should they violate patient confidentiality and privacy. Essentially, the credentialing process allows students access to the hospital ED, within their scope of credentialing (i.e., no patient care) and to patient interactions. Approval of participant observation from the hospital administration was easier to obtain (even with HIPAA concerns) than it was to obtain that approval from IRB which maintained that human subjects in that space had a higher right to privacy, even though no PHI was being collected or disclosed.

Both RDB and JWW have interacted with the local university IRB many times and have both developed a strategy that if a protocol is reviewed by IRB and returned for changes two times, then a phone call with an IRB reviewer is needed. If a third review of an IRB protocol still leads to a return of the protocol requesting further modifications, we feel that this is an appropriate time for a face-to-face meeting with IRB leadership (manager and/or chair). Our participant observation protocol required a series of those meetings.

In meetings with IRB managers and directors, they have expressed their understanding of the hospital credentialing process and clearance but focus on their legal considerations surrounding the 45 Code of Federal Regulations 46 (45 CFR 46) known as the Protection of Human Subjects (OHRP 2016). Much of the responsibility for local/university institutional review boards place heavy emphasis on protecting organizations from any perceived or potential violations of 45 CFR 46. In our estimation, this focus on law does not always align with the initial goal of human subjects protections laid out in sentinel papers like the Belmont Report (OHRP 2010) which was originally to ensure that individuals had autonomy, respect for privacy, and that no undue harm was committed by researchers on research participants. We have sometimes been surprised at how little the local IRB is concerned with some projects and the minimal amount of review and documented consent required for research participants in some medical drug studies, or studies on refugee prior trauma—but how much review and documentation is required surrounding sensitive subjects or perceived sensitive areas where multiple federal laws may intertwine (HIPAA and 45 CFR 46) to create an environment of concern for risk exposure and legal liability to the organization but not necessarily any risk, or very minimal risk, to the research participant. For example, we maintain that if PHI is not being collected, stored, analyzed and that there is no specific intervention being applied to one group compared to another, the risk to human subjects is likely low. However, we have struggled to gain approval for the required work of "hanging out" to do thick descriptions that anthropologists must do and to convey to IRB representatives how minimal the risk is to those around the researcher during their time conducting participant observation.

There is dual concern surrounding 45 CFR 46 and HIPAA liability exposure for the organization (again compare this to the initial goal of IRB to protect actual or potential research participants) and there is also added concern and confusion surrounding the types of projects we are conducting as medical anthropologists directly in a clinical space. By definition, our interest as applied researchers is to find ways that anthropological questions and methods can address actual healthcare and medical problems. Thus, we utilize mixed methods and ask questions that are difficult to frame as purely social or purely medical. Our local IRB, however, is divided into essentialist social and medical divisions. We have witnessed several of our studies being reassigned back and forth between each IRB multiple times. For example, an ongoing study with patients that present to the ED with sickle cell disease shifts between a few data collection spaces (chapter 8). For example, we may monitor traditional patient throughput and health services–related outcomes such as ED length of stay, hospital admission rate, pain control on a visual analog scale, return visits over a year, drug dose, type of drug, and drug delivery method. At the same time, we may also interview patients with sickle cell disease about their experiences in the ED compared to the infusion center to better understand suffering and stigma. As most anthropologists, a lot of the project time might also be spent simply hanging out with sickle cell disease patient care providers (hematologists) and talking with ED staff about their attitudes regarding patients requiring high doses of opioid pain medicine. Our goal in that work might be to search for patterns of care delivery that lead to stigma and suffering or to test potential specific interventions that decrease stigma and suffering. Is this social science or medicine?

We believe the binary division is false and that our work specifically moves in between the social and the medical, offering a valuable approach to solving medical questions in which the same solution or type of solutions have been reproduced over time simply because the questions asked are limited (e.g., focus on another biomedical intervention to decrease pain in sickle cell disease patients instead of eliciting driving factors for care seeking and unraveling the context of suffering). Sometimes, we also are not sure if our study protocols should be submitted to the social science or the medical IRB.

Adams et al. (2014) described the value of anthropological methods in current global health research, specifically emphasizing the "slow research" approach that anthropologists take to the culture and place of interest. In an era where consultants, development workers, or public health officials often swoop in and swoop out of an area with a predetermined question in mind on arrival, the deep roots and context of place and people is lost or not part of interpretation. We echo the emphasis on "deep hanging out" made popular by Clifford Geertz (1988) and continue to find value in the anthropological approach to developing hypotheses in which the questions are not always predetermined but may arise from long periods of participant observation.

We still assign the 1978 article by Arthur Kleinman et al. that outlines mismatches in explanatory models of disease and illness as well as the basic issues challenging healthcare (expense, unsatisfied patients). When students read this article, we ask, what did you notice? Most point out that the article is over 40 years old. The students (especially the medical residents who see patients every day) then point out and agree that nothing has changed or things may have gotten worse in healthcare since publication of this article. In other words, approaching problems in healthcare the same way we always have is not working. Our belief is that interdisciplinary approaches outlined in this book bring a patient-centered approach to problem-solving, hardwire that into the next generation of physicians while simultaneously addressing contemporary problems in healthcare that are not just of theoretical concern to the social scientist but of actual praxes concern to the physician and medical system. Thus, we must find a way to do participant observation in healthcare settings—otherwise, medical anthropologists remain arms distance, or paraclinical, instead of clinical in their approaches to medical problem-solving and essentially become potentially irrelevant to colleagues in medicine from the onset.

The IRB staff considers the ED waiting room a space with an inherent expectation of privacy. We have considered the possibility of HIPAA waivers (USFRI). HIPAA waivers can be utilized in cases where some PHI is observed, often in a screening process. In other words, if we are studying a new blood pressure medication, we might look at the track board (list of active patients) in the electronic medical record and identify those in the ED with high blood pressure. A RA might then approach that patient to ask further questions to consider inclusion and exclusion criteria as well as patient interest in study participation. During this "prescreening" process, the RA has accessed private information of large numbers of patients to review blood pressure and to find a patient for further review of inclusion and exclusion criteria for a specific study protocol. HIPAA waivers for this prescreening activity are routinely granted. In other words, "hanging out" in a virtual waiting room is acceptable while "hanging out" in the physical waiting room is considered a violation of the expected privacy when entering a hospital environment, even though a student or RA will view and access much more PHI in the virtual waiting room prescreening space than a physical space.

Our interest is in moving to a place of "hanging out" physically where we really do not need students to know any specific patient details or PHI. However, engrained logics of physicality limit understanding of private data access and where real privacy is potentially violated (with waivered permission) at scale (electronically).

Obtaining signed HIPAA waivers is also complicated by IRB, which requires that potential participants can be consented in privacy without the influence of any medical staff. The required HIPAA language and informed consent documents by the IRB would also mean that participants would have to read through a five-page document before they could be observed. These requirements make it impossible for students to obtain proper consent and HIPAA waivers and observe, without disrupting the flow of the ED. Additionally, such long forms seem to be overkill for the risk versus the cost to very ill patients and, again, actually provide research staff with more PHI than is requested or needed for participant observation.

Further complicating the study approval process are the separate applications for studies from each institution. The study approval process at the hospital has a series of documents where other departments, such as nursing, must approve studies before they are considered by the OCR. Specifically, a study protocol is submitted first to IRB, next IRB sends the study protocol to the hospital OCR. The hospital does not have its own IRB and instead utilizes the university/local IRB or a central IRB. A central IRB is a national level commercial entity (e.g., wIRB) in which investigators or study sponsors pay large fees for study review. Given that most of our medical anthropology and class studies are unfunded, we utilize the local/university IRB. The hospital is an approved designated site of the local IRB. The designated site must first clear the study before the study protocol moves forward the IRB review process.

The hospital OCR initiates their review of the protocol, focusing on hospital feasibility and hospital risk/exposure. After changes are made based on hospital OCR review, the protocol is then assigned to the affected and impacted areas of the hospital—for instance, a study that enrolls patients with appendicitis (an infection of the appendix) might need approval from hospital workers (usually nurse manager or nursing director) in the ED, the OR, and the PACU (postanesthesia care unit). An education plan for the study is also required in which study staff must outline ways in which they will spend time with each impacted hospital area to discuss study goals and any staff roles as well as how the study will affect clinical operations and patient care. After approval by appropriate nursing leadership and hospital OCR, the study can be cleared by the designated site (the hospital) and continue moving forward in IRB review. Often during hospital review, many of the same documents submitted to IRB are required to be resubmitted or submitted with changes to the hospital (again, thanks to a recent merging of the USF and TGH research offices, many of these administrative burdens are finally being addressed at the time of this writing). As with the credentialing process, the study approval process and documents have also had frequent changes of which we are often unaware. Despite the designated site having to approve any research done there, as the IRB process continues, we often find that both institutions often do not agree on what are acceptable procedures.

There are multiple categories of review that can be requested of IRB. If a study does not access PHI and presents no harm, the study may meet exempt status under the Common Rule which outlines those studies evaluating courses or classes, surveys, interviews, or observations of public behaviors with no PHI and no inclusion of prisoners or children may be exempt. QI projects are also not research (i.e., there is no experimental intervention) and are exempt from IRB consideration since there is no human research. We have not been able to meet the standards for exemption in our "research" projects, given the higher level of privacy expectations (e.g., greater than a public space) that IRB feels patients have in a hospital setting.

The next category of IRB review is expedited. Expedited review can be completed by an assigned IRB reviewer and then approved by the IRB chair or director. We have been able to obtain expedited IRB review for our research studies with narrow focus or specific hypotheses (e.g., does exercise help patients with diabetes control hemoglobin A1C levels?). But, again, we have not been able to reach expedited approval to conduct participant observation in the ED. The final, and most rigorous, category of IRB review is full board meeting and full review. This level of review is usually reserved for studies with a specific intervention or experimental group, and we have not taken any of our studies to this level of review at this time. We feel if the participant observation, hanging out type of work, were to move to full IRB review, we would be required to engage in a written consent process with every patient and every person present in the ED. In other words, we understand the concerns raised by IRB and under 46 CFR 45, there is likely not a clear way this type of research can easily be integrated into the ED as part of a "research" project, but this does not mean that participant observation cannot be done in other ways (discussed below) to still inform applied medical anthropology in the clinical setting.

Another issue, particularly for undergraduate student thesis projects, has been the length of time necessary to get a project through the many levels of approval at the hospital and through IRB review. Initially, our goal was for students to move a project from idea to prospectus during the first part of the semester and then submit the study to IRB at the end of the semester (as the final capstone) with IRB approval the next semester allowing the student to begin conducting research at that time. However, the turnaround time for these projects often took the entire next semester. In addition, having the student listed as PI was not ideal for a few reasons. First, the student as PI is not a known researcher to IRB, with no formed relationships or history of trust developed with that staff or the hospital. This may create a higher standard or increased level of scrutiny since a student may not fully understand the importance of human subjects protection or the need to not commit protocol deviations (or the regulatory steps necessary in the event of a protocol deviation). Second, students simply have many competing obligations and shifting emphasis on what and when something is important leading to delays in turnaround of requested IRB or hospital documents. Finally, as researchers with a serious interest in helping solve ongoing problems in medicine, a model of student projects with that student as PI was not very impactful.

Instead, we have moved to a set of longitudinal projects in which the faculty (JWW and RDB) are the PIs. This allows the faculty to develop long-term projects that can be completed over multiple semesters, not just one, adding data in a serial manner as a student joins the project. Each semester, the student who joins an ongoing project can create an addendum to an already approved IRB protocol that carves out space of interest and intellectual property for that student. For example, if we want to examine cultural and structural variation in hemoglobin A1C control in diabetics, one student might spend time asking about time spent exercising in good and poorly controlled diabetics, while another might compare a group of Southeast Asian patients to a group of African American patients. Each student though will maintain some shared interview questions and collect a core set of similar data, adding to a growing data set over time. However, an IRB amendment allows that student to add some specific data collection elements (e.g., number of hours spent exercising per week). That student can write about the overall project and then analyze the data they collected, framing the analysis within their own question, but also considering all the data for context. RDB and JWW are then able to grow the data set and consider broader patterns and help guide future students in directions that might address gaps in the longitudinal work.

However, even in the case of research projects that are deemed acceptable, we are often required to use the lengthy written consent forms. This process seems ethically questionable for patients who are in an ED as many of those patients have a low reading level (fourth grade). Standard written consent forms are an example of where we feel that emphasis by IRBs on liability exposure instead of appropriateness for patients is evident. Lengthy written consent forms at a high reading level are inappropriate for ED patients and out of alignment with current estimates of health literacy. Many patients have a reading level estimated to be between fourth and sixth grade, but many approved consent forms are above that level. The recommended consent form provided by our local IRB may be too difficult for ED patients, especially during an acute care episode. RDB has modified the consent form, and it has been approved by our IRB for use in our firearm injury study (chapter 11), providing an example where we feel that more human subjects protection was needed than that required by the local IRB. In other words, at times, we are surprised by the amount of scrutiny paid to our qualitative, deidentified, semi-structured interviews in the context of clinical drug trials that may receive less oversight. At other times, we are worried about our most vulnerable patient populations—some of which have not been easy to access by other researchers (e.g., patients with lower levels of education or limited English proficiency, patients experiencing acute withdrawal or overdose, or patients that have been shot)—and we have built in further consent language and requirements to meet a higher ethical bar when working with those specific patient groups.

QI AND APPLIED CLINICAL MEDICAL ANTHROPOLOGY

The triple aim paradigm (IHI) is shifting medicine from a fee-for-service model to a value of service model. Thus, emphases on QI and patient safety have become critically strategic for hospital administration to protect thin profit margins that could be eroded by low benchmark scores on quality outcomes. We have found that alignment of our projects with ongoing QI projects at the hospital garner more attention and may provide more value to our hospital partners than investigator-initiated research questions. For example, a project that examines patient experiences who come to the ED, wait for a long period of time, and leave without being seen is of much greater interest to hospital administrators since the percent of patients that leave without being seen in the ED is publicly reportable and tied to revenue generation as this represents a significant patient safety concern as those that leave without being seen may come back to the ED sicker and requiring more complex, and expensive, medical care.

In addition, QI projects are not human subjects research, even though many of the methods and approaches are similar—that is, a question or topic area is considered, a literature review is conducted, consideration of benchmark or current process is done, a potential intervention or observation period is planned, and post-intervention analysis is then conducted. However, QI is not human subjects research because the goal of QI is to implement or maintain an already identified best practice. In other words, you know the outcome you want, the outcome that is best for your patients, and the goal is to find ways to help the institution or provider reach that outcome. Many institutions have created guidelines for whether a project should be considered research or QI. Figure 4.1 is the set of guidelines provided by the USF IRB to help investigators determine which type of project their protocol is considered.

Thus, for several reasons, we now prioritize QI projects whenever possible. These projects have higher stakeholder buy-in (the hospital partner is more interested in the outcomes), do not involve human subjects research permission (and, thus, require fewer formal approvals), are not in the scope of 46 CFR 45, and allow for broader ability of students to observe the ED within the framework of the ongoing QI project, and the results are more likely to be incorporated into hospital procedures. The QI format speaks to hospital administrators and other staff who are concerned with improving both patient experience and publicly reportable hospital throughput and patient outcome statistics. While we still obtain informed verbal consent for our interviews, and abide by HIPAA, conducting QI projects means we do not have to use the lengthy IRB-required forms and can use verbal consent scripts written at

COMPARISON: CHARACTERISTICS OF HUMAN SUBJECT RESEARCH VS. QUALITY IMPROVEMENT, PROGRAM EVALUATION, OR CLASS/STUDENT PROJECTS Determining whether a project requires IRB review depends on whether it constitutes research involving human subjects (first column). Please contact the USF IRB Office (813-974-5638) with any questions or for assistance in making a determination.

	HUMAN SUBJECT RESEARCH	QUALITY IMPROVEMENT	PROGRAM EVALUATION	CLASS / STUDENT PROJECT
INTENT	Project is to develop or contribute to generalizable knowledge (e.g., testing hypotheses)	Intent of project is to improve a practice or process within a particular institution or ensure it confirms with expected norms	Intent of project is to improve a specific program, only to provide information for and about the setting in which it is conducted	Intent of project is to provide an educational experience about the research process or methods
MOTIVATION FOR PROJECT	Project occurs in large part as a result of individual professional goals and requirements (e.g., seeking tenure; obtaining grants; completing a thesis or dissertation)	Project occurs regardless of whether individual(s) conducting it may benefit professionally from conducting the project	Project not initiated by the evaluator and occurs regardless of whether individual(s) conducting it may benefit professionally from conducting the project	Project occurs as part of assigned course/class work or a requirement of an educational program in order to learn a new technique or pass a course/fulfill an assignment
DESIGN	Designed to develop or contribute to generalizable knowledge; may involve randomization of individuals to different treatments, regimens, or processes; novel research ideas supported by literature search	Not designed to develop or contribute to generalizable knowledge; generally does not involve randomization to different practices or processes	Not designed to develop or contribute to generalizable knowledge; does not involve randomization of individuals, but may involve comparison of variations in programs	Not designed to develop or contribute to generalizable knowledge; design is often an example or template provided by a professor or course book
MANDATE	Activities not mandated by institution or program	Activity mandated by the institution or clinic as part of its operations	Activity mandated by the program, usually its funder, as part of its operations	Activity mandated by regularly assigned coursework or educational program
EFFECT ON PROGRAM OR PRACTICE EVALUATED	Findings of the study are not expected to directly or immediately affect institutional or programmatic practice	Findings of the study are expected to directly affect institutional practice and identify corrective action(s) needed	Findings of the evaluation are expected to directly affect the conduct of the program and identify improvements	Findings of project are not expected to directly affect the program; the project will mainly generate raw data, not generalizable knowledge
SUBJECT POPULATION	Usually involves a subset of individuals; universal participation of an entire clinic, program, or department is not expected; generally, statistical justification for sample size is used to ensure endpoints can be met	Information on all or most receiving a particular treatment or undergoing a particular practice or process expected to be included; exclusion of information from some individuals significantly affects conclusions	Information on all or most participants within or affected by receiving a particular treatment or undergoing a particular practice or process expected to be used; exclusion of information from some individuals significantly affects conclusions	Can either include all, most, or a subset of individuals; statistical justification may be used in the context to understand the process of subject selection; however, recruitment often utilizes convenience sampling
BENEFITS	Participants may or may not benefit directly. If there is benefit to participants, it is often incidental or delayed	Participants expected to benefit directly from the activities	No benefit to participants expected; evaluation concentrates on program improvements or whether the program should continue	Participants may or may not benefit directly; benefit is primarily for the investigator conducting project for his/her own knowledge or fulfillment of educational requirements
DISSEMINATION OF RESULTS	Intent to publish or present generally presumed at the outset of project as part of professional expectations, obligations; dissemination of information usually occurs in research/scientific publications, grant proposals, or other research/ scientific forum; results expected to develop or contribute to generalizable knowledge by filling a gap in scientific knowledge or supporting, refining, or refuting results from other research studies	Intent to publish or present generally not presumed at the outset of the project; dissemination of information often does not occur beyond the institution evaluated; dissemination of information may occur in quality improvement publications/fora; when published or presented to a wider audience, the intent is to suggest potentially effective models, strategies, assessment tools or provide benchmarks or base rates rather than to develop or contribute to generalizable knowledge	Intent to publish or present generally presumed at the outset of the project; dissemination of information to program stakeholders and participants; may be publicly posted (e.g., website) to ensure transparency of results; when published or presented to a wider audience, the intent is to suggest potentially effective models, strategies, assessment tools or provide benchmarks or base rates rather than to develop or contribute to generalizable knowledge	No intent to present or publish results beyond the classroom, campus, or educational program; any presentations, posters, or publishing (such as on USF website) is simply to document completed work/raw data for educational or programmatic requirements and/or to obtain experience

Copyright, UT Arlington. Modified and used with permission from UT Arlington. 11/3/2015

Figure 4.1 *Source*: Reproduced from USF BULLSIRB Site (2021) From UT Arlington, November 1, 2015.

a fifth-grade reading level. Focusing on QI projects has also allowed us to answer important scholarly questions without disrupting the flow of the ED and inconveniencing patients and staff with a lengthy written consent process.

FUNDING

Up to the present, there has not been any formal funding for our projects. The Honors College has covered the stipend for Wilson, and initially the Anthropology Department was content that the FTE (student credit hours) for our courses be assigned to them. Later, as university-wide funding cuts have hit departments, Anthropology has moved to requesting partial funding from the Honors College to compensate for Baer's teaching of students under the Honors College label. However, more budget cuts are anticipated, and we are concerned that the entire financial burden has fallen to the Honors College. It is not clear to us that this funding mechanism is sustainable for the two undergraduate courses.

SCALING UP

A final challenge has been scaling up. The demand for courses of this type is huge; usually over 100 students apply for 15 spots in the Research Experience in Patient Provider Interaction class. The dean of the Honors College has encouraged us to scale up. However, an attempt to admit more students (23) was not successful. Class cohesion—which is integral in a course that demands a group research project be carried out during a 15-week semester—seemed to suffer. As such, we have found ourselves growing the project vertically—expanding into the residents' training at the USF medical school, as opposed to creating more classes for undergraduates, beyond the basic hospital class and the thesis class. Ideally, horizontal expansion would also be possible if other dyads were motivated—or at least other physicians in different spaces. For example, one model we have considered is a hub-and-spoke model in which we serve as the center of a course, meeting with a large group of students while also still maintaining their own pod of 10 to 15 students that will work in the ED, while a family physician, pediatric physician, internal medicine physician, surgeon, and OB physician could also each take 10 to 15 students to accommodate and create parallel clinical experiences. To date, we have not identified other physicians motivated to do similar work to that of the first author with undergraduate students in their own clinical spaces. However, academic physicians have shown interest in similar programs for medical students and residents, allowing these vertical expansion attempts more success. And the advantage of working with medical students and residents is that they are already credentialed, eliminating a huge paperwork processing activity for our graduate assistant. We find ourselves in a quandary as to how to expand the undergraduate activities, given that we cannot clone ourselves. So, our current thoughts are to encourage others who are interested in these approaches to find appropriate team members and broaden the endeavors in that fashion.

Chapter 5

Expanding the Vision

Working with Residents and Medical Students

In the fall of 2018, we were contacted by the internal medicine residency program director at the University of South Florida (USF) (Kellee Oller, MD) who was familiar with our previous work with undergraduate students on topics related to patient experience. Dr. Oller had a place in the schedule for a wellness workshop (focusing on better sleep and other approaches to the stresses of residency), which in the past had not gone well (mandated curriculum changes to improve wellness are controversial and still evolving area meant to combat an ongoing physician burnout epidemic). The residents wanted something more practical and useful than the material covered during the wellness workshop the previous year. The hospital had also been talking with the Department of Internal Medicine residency program about the need to improve patient experiences scores related to patient encounters between internal medicine residents and admitted hospitalized patients.

The Centers for Medicare and Medicaid Services requires hospitals to administer the Hospital Consumer Assessment of Healthcare Providers and Systems (HCAHPS—pronounced "H-CAPS"). The survey is a national standardized survey with reimbursement implications for hospitals performing below (loss of Medicare revenue) or above (additional Medicare revenue) the mean (HCAHPS, Retrieved 6/21). Resident-patient encounters account for a large volume of patient encounters across the hospital and thus are a significant driver of overall HCAHP scores.

The internal medicine residency program director specifically requested that we spend time with the internal medicine residents in the format of a two-day workshop covering issues related to patient experience and potential ways that the overall experience of patients in the hospital might be improved.

We (RDB and JWW) considered the material we covered in our semester-long undergraduate course but were constrained by the limits of the possibilities of a two-day workshop format. Instead, we decided to focus on issues that we had already identified in the undergraduate course (gaps in provider and patient expectations and explanatory models) and to emphasize the methodology we used to bring those issues quickly to light during the undergraduate experience—patient shadowing. The workshop took place with second-year medical residents. Second-year residents have completed college, medical school, and are in their second year of an intensive three-year physician training program. We felt that this was still an opportune time to intervene and interject the potentiality of a patient-centered gaze.

METHODS

All the second-year internal medicine residents were required to attend the workshop for the purpose of exploring the issue of patient experience and patient satisfaction. Before meeting on day 1, we distributed a pretest. When that had been completed, we sent two articles to all the participants—one on participant observation (Crane and Angrosino 1992) and the other about differences in patient-provider perspectives (Kleinman et al. 1978).

The first year we ran the workshop, it was well received, and we were invited back in 2019 to run the workshop again. Based on feedback from the inaugural workshop participants, we removed the Crane and Angrosino chapter about participant observation. To ensure relevance, we substituted the term "participant observation" for "patient shadowing" (even though the method is essentially the same). Instead of the chapter on participant observation, we included an article covering structural determinants of healthcare and published by a team of physicians and physician-anthropologists in the *New England Journal of Medicine* as part of a multi-issue series on social determinants in healthcare using clinical vignettes to demonstrate relevance of the encounters and the assessment of structural determinants more directly to practicing physicians (Seymour et al. 2018). The combination of the Kleinman et al. (1978) and the Seymour et al. (2018) perspectives allows residents to specifically develop ways to integrate structural competency as well as ways to close the gap between patient and provider explanatory models of disease and illness.

In a two-hour session on day 1, JWW and RDB reviewed the assigned readings with the group of approximately 40 residents. Next, we gave the residents their assignment for day 2. Each resident would spend time conducting patient shadowing (participant observation in a patient room) for four to five hours the next morning after being assigned an appropriate patient by the program director (i.e., a patient admitted to the university hospitalist teaching service). After lunch on day 2, there was a two-hour debrief meeting with

JWW and RDB in which residents shared their patient shadowing experiences. In addition, a video was shown which dramatizes the experience of an English-speaking patient in a hospital Emergency Department (ED) attempting to obtain care for a sick infant. In the video (a public service announcement created by the Texas Association of Healthcare Interpreters, TAHIT 2010), the mother of an infant with a very high temperature is the only native English speaker and becomes more irate and agitated as the ED staff continue to try and have the woman calm down and complete bureaucratic registration processes (TAHIT 2010).

The pre- and posttests were used to determine changes in perspective and possible influence of the workshop on resident approaches to the overall patient experience during hospitalization. Among the residents, 37 completed the pretest and 28 responded to the posttest, both of which asked for open-ended responses. These responses were coded by themes by two coders who first coded independently. The coders then compared and discussed differences in coding to insure inter-coder reliability of coding.

RESULTS

We wanted to first explore two important issues: (1) What are the patient's expectations of a hospital visit? (2) How does the patient learn about what to expect? The residents learned that their impact and the overall influence of treating providers and staff on the overall patient care plan was less than they realized (43% pre, 39% post). In addition, workshop participants' understanding of patient perspectives was based on personal experience with themselves or family members (52% pre, 61% post). Understanding of patient expectations also changed; residents learned that patients highly valued being treated with respect (37% pre, 57% post), feeling better during the hospital stay (22% pre, 57% post), and effective communication with the patient (35% pre, 57% post) were key issues.

Next, we addressed the patient's perception of communication and collaboration among the medical team of nursing, physicians, staff, and patients. What does the patient understand about the individual roles of each person entering the room? What is the patient's idea of the optimal model of care?

Initially, only some residents felt that patients might be confused about who comes in the room (44%) and thought patients were receiving adequate amounts of communication (67%). Overall, pre-workshop responses were very physician centric and defensive. The posttest responses were more patient centric and demonstrated better recognition of the patient's perspective. Compared to the pretest, residents realized that patients do not know who is coming in the room (71% posttest compared to 44% pretest). In the posttest, only 25% of residents felt that patients had experienced adequate communication with their providers. Residents also mentioned the lack of communication between treatment staff which they observed directly and were frustrated with the discontinuity of treatment for the patient.

Many times, the residents witnessed a consultant physician (e.g., cardiologist) relay a care plan that was in conflict or direct opposition to another consultant (e.g., gastroenterologist) or the primary care team (internal medicine). In addition, the residents witnessed the primary care team ask the patient, on multiple occasions, what the consultants were planning to do, as the primary care team had been unable to directly discuss patient care with the consultants and hoped to glean that information from the patient. The best practice for team communication is to conduct interdisciplinary rounds as discussed by physician and now patient experience leader, James Merlino, from the Cleveland Clinic in his book *Service Fanatics* (2014) and by other patient safety and best practice organizations, including the Institute for Healthcare Improvement (IHI). Ideally, interdisciplinary (or multidisciplinary) rounding would include multiple physician specialties along with nursing, social work, pharmacy, physical therapy, dietary, and any other support staff involved in the patient's care. However, timing and implementation of multidisciplinary rounding across physician service lines have remained limited at most institutions. This speaks to the lack of patient centeredness in how most hospital organizations still operate.

For example, the residents noted that phlebotomist (staff that obtains blood samples) enters the room very early in the morning (usually before 6:00 a.m.), awakens the patient, and obtains samples for several diagnostic tests that often have low utility to repeat frequently, and may have been done the day before (but order sets from residents gain inertia, leading to daily repeat labs on automatic pilot). The lack of ability to execute multidiscipline physician rounds and timing of blood draws are two excellent examples of the current design of a healthcare system that is physician centered. Given the competing, and differing across specialties, demands of the OR, clinic, morning rounds, teaching time, and night shifts, each specialty struggles to coordinate group rounding. Labs are done for the convenience of rounding teams, not for the value of the patient. Currently, most hospital systems have attempted to redesign and implement lean approaches (completing steps in care that add value for the patient while attempting to remove steps that do not add direct patient value and are considered "waste"). However, the design of this current healthcare system is rooted in deep medical culture that may take years to change or require further incentivization to tilt from good recommendations to urgent changes.

Residents also observed that most people who enter a patient room do not introduce themselves. The residents observed that patients become frustrated that they did not know who staff was, or what the role of different members in their care team would be in their hospital management. In addition, conversations with patients demonstrated that many patients had little idea about why particular procedures or diagnostic testing was being done during their hospital stay.

Posttest data demonstrated that residents were concerned that patients get overwhelmed and frustrated because of lack of communication and lack of clarity about who is in the room and why.

The third topic we explored in our pre- and post-workshop question design was factors that contribute to the patient's ability to manage care outside of the hospital before the admission and after the hospital discharge. SES, health literacy/knowledge, and social support were seen both pre and post as key contributing factors to care. However, in the posttest, additional factors were noted, including language, time, and culture/race/gender:

> An array of factors including social, economic, mental, and physical [affect a patient's ability to manage their care]. We can make the most wonderful plan however if the patient is unable to follow such recommendations for any reason, then there is no actual help being given for that problem.—Anonymous Second-Year Resident

> Patients need to understand what disease they have and how it reflects or leads to their symptoms. They need to understand how medicine and prescribed treatment will cure their disease and treat their illness. They all need to have social support and resources necessary to be able to care for themselves.—Anonymous Second-Year Resident

Next, we addressed how patients think the relationships in the hospital affect the overall delivery of their care (patient-physician relationship, patient care team relationship). Previous work on patient experience (Press 2006) has demonstrated that a patient's perspective on the status of their relationship with the care team and among the care team itself are key drivers in the amount of trust a patient has for the organization and physician, directly impacting the ability to carry out a treatment plan.

In the pretest responses, 89% of residents said that how the patient perceives care may be more important than whether the standard of care is being met.

Other pretest responses were like those of the posttest (better relationship equals better care, or that there is a direct relationship between relationship and care, and how patients need to trust the physician 79%). Communication issues affecting the physician-patient relationship were noted in pre- and posttest responses, but only in the posttest was trust (18%) mentioned:

> The better patient-physician relationship can aid better medical condition understanding for the patient and will likely have better outcomes.—Anonymous Second-Year Resident

> When the patient has a good relationship with the physician and care team, the care the patient received is often improved. The patient will likely be more honest with the medical team (both about positive areas and areas with need for improvement), and the patient may feel more comfortable talking to the medical team to provide a full description of his/her symptoms, concerns and needs, which should positively impact the delivery of care. Even if the care is excellent, if the patient does not have a positive relationship with the physician and/or care team, the perceived delivery of care can be harmed.—Anonymous Second-Year Resident

However, overall, there was a shift to understanding that patients know when they are receiving poor care, and the onus isn't on just the patient (e.g., not just patients thinking things are good or bad).

The next question on the pre- and post-workshop questionnaire asked, how much does a patient understand of what their care team tells them? How much do they remember? Similar percentages of pre- and posttest responses felt that patient understands some of the delivered information but often does not remember the information (41% pre, 43% post). However, in the posttest, 36% of residents gave a response not mentioned at all in the pretest responses—that how much the patient knows/remembers depends on the communication and type of language used (indicating a recognition that building trust with the patient may lead to better understanding of delivered medical information and the care plan). Additional factors mentioned in the posttest included patient characteristics and what the patient feels are important:

> This varies greatly depending on the patient, as well as how their care team explains things to them. They will often only remember what they perceived to be the most important points to them, based on their priorities or values.—Anonymous Second-Year Resident

> The patient often understands very little of the information that is given to them due to the vast jargon and speed at which the information is given. If we had more time and were able to more slowly relay the information, it may help with better understanding.—Anonymous Second-Year Resident

Residents were then asked, what are the most positive things about a patient's experience at the hospital? Residents initially felt the most important factor was quality of care (73%). Most studies demonstrate that patients are not able to evaluate their quality of care and instead use proxy measures (e.g., room cleanliness) to instead attempt to assess quality (Press 2006, Merlino 2015). After completion of patient shadowing, only 25% of residents still felt that quality of care was an important issue to patients. However, in line with previously published studies, results of the posttest demonstrated that the residents recognized that quality of staff (including nursing, custodial staff, as well as physicians) was important and that response increased from 32% in the pretest to 54% in the posttest. The residents recognized that patients included custodians, nurses, and other support staff and not just physicians as part of the care team:

> The staff. That was repeated over and over again during our feedback sessions and by the patient I spent time with. They really enjoyed the kindness and positivity of everyone. The accessibility of staff as well. My patient in particular felt very comfortable, their guests did as well.—Anonymous Second-Year Resident

> Some of the most positive things about a patient's experience at TGH are the quality of the physicians/care team, access to specialists, and ability to have almost all procedures/imaging completed within the hospital. Another aspect that can be a positive or a negative depending on the patient is being at a training hospital where multiple people will see the patient which can lead to more information being shared with the team which helps to provide thorough care.—Anonymous Second-Year Resident

After considering what residents felt were important positive aspects of the hospital stay to patients, we then focused on the most negative things about a patient's experience. When considering negative aspects of the patient experience, communication went from 30% to 57% (pre/posttest) and was seen as the most negative aspect of the patient experience. In the pre-shadowing assessment, 35% of residents thought that "poor care" would be the most negative aspect of the patient experience. However, poor care decreased from 35% in the pre-workshop to not even being mentioned in the post-workshop questionnaire. Wait times were also considered as a negative aspect of the care encounter and went from 35% to 25%. In addition, frequency of tests/interruptions/lack of sleep for patients were not mentioned in the pretest but were noted by 29% of residents in the post survey:

> Some of the most negative things about a patient's experience at [the hospital] include difficulty with communication between the primary physician/specialists/care team which can be frustrating/confusing, delays in ability to have a

> procedure performed due to scheduling/high volume, being frequently awoken, and frequent lab draws.—Anonymous Second-Year Resident

> Doctors coming to visit at their own time, when asking for a medication it takes 2 hours for it to come back, the food is hit or miss, and at times not knowing why certain things are being done to them in the hospital (i.e., lab draws).—Anonymous Second-Year Resident

The next questions were not on the pre-workshop questionnaire, as they focused on the value of the workshop. We asked the residents questions about what they learned from the readings and class discussion before their observation. The key issues mentioned by 54% of the participants were the difference between disease (the physician's model) and illness (the patient's model of what is happening to them). In addition, the need to address illness and/or cultural beliefs was also noted by 36% of respondents. However, 7% noted that they already knew these things:

> There are a lot of cultural beliefs that can be overlooked. It is important to take the time to address the illness whenever possible.—Anonymous Second-Year Resident

> The major take home for me were the differences between illness and disease, and the questions needed to help elicit this. I knew, for the most part, most of the negative things that come with an inpatient stay, but I did not know the extent of them and the toll it takes on every patient.—Anonymous Second-Year Resident

> Communication is crucial—no one doubts that—but it's also very hard to effectively achieve.—Anonymous Second-Year Resident

> I learned that to truly become a better physician one must treat not only the disease but illness of a patient.—Anonymous Second-Year Resident

> I learned that disease is not equal to illness and that patient's experience both and come to the hospital to get treatment for both. Sadly, physicians are trained in treating diseases and sometimes that patients' expectations don't align with the current healthcare model.—Anonymous Second-Year Resident

Finally, we asked the resident participants what they had learned from their patient observations. Thirty nine percent of the anonymous second-year resident comments addressed communication:

- Frustrating that physicians can't spend a lot of time talking to the patients.

- Recognize that communication is important.
- Need to actually practice patient-centered care instead of just saying we do.
- Need to better understand disease versus illness, empower patients, how slow things move for patients.
- Need to be able to communicate and utilize nursing better. Important to consider patient concerns and not take things personally.
- Disservice to patients that we have no time to communicate with them.
- Chronically ill patients have a lot of experience and their experiences should help inform patient-centered care.

Twenty five percent of the residents also noted the importance of patient-centered care/understanding of the patient perspective/experience. Eleven percent of the residents felt that patient shadowing was an interesting/good experience and was an out-of-the-box training.

Eleven percent did not find the workshop useful:

- Patient had no complaints. Residents know all about communication barriers and long wait times. Was condescending.
- Understands the purpose but doesn't think it should be for second-year residents, and would be better for med students, interns, or attending physicians. Residents learn this in med school already but attending physicians may be too far removed or may not have learned this in school.
- Residents don't know how to implement change within the system, so that would be a more helpful exercise, to teach residents how to plan a strategy to get the administration to make changes.
- Already knew everything.
- Want a survey with choices or a box for an input of ideas for them to decide what type of retreat or workshop the majority wants.

In summary, we feel this brief medical resident training was extremely effective. Specific changes in perspective were seen in the areas of increased understanding of the differences between the patient's and physician's perspectives, as well as the importance of communication in effective patient care. We have also been invited to continue the workshop each spring.

While a minority of the residents felt they already know it all (a perspective not supported by their low patient experience scores, the reason the workshop was initiated), we do agree with some of the statements of this group. Residency is rather late for a focus on the importance of the patient experience; it needs to come much earlier, as in our class for premedical undergraduates and the experiences we are constructing for medical students.

Residents observed specific events that they would like to change (early lab draws, lack of team communication, low use of interpreter services) but did not feel confident in their knowledge of how to make system changes. In subsequent years, we will invite hospital administration to our debriefing sessions and have begun working with the internal medicine residency program leadership to begin assisting residents to develop change management strategies. We hope this will lead to the development of more action plans based on the residents' experiences in the workshop.

Finally, the perspective of the residents that this training belongs in the medical school curriculum is one we strongly share. Our initial goal was to teach the material in our premed course in a medical school context, but there were several institutional barriers to this. However, at the urging of our premedical students who are now in medical school at our institution, who also felt that all their medical school colleagues should share the experiences they had in our class, we were invited to do an elective experience in spring 2020 for the first-year medical students at the USF Morsani Medical School. Medical students have small amount of elective time in the doctoring course (which teaches what being a physician is about) and our workshop (which we will base on the residents' workshop) is now one of the electives they can choose. For spring 2020, we had six students signed up to participate in a patient shadowing participant observation experience for the semester. This was delayed that spring by hospital Covid-19 restrictions and is planned for reimplementation in fall 2021.

Based on our experiences, we highly recommend patient shadowing for medical personnel at all levels. To our knowledge, only the Cleveland Clinic has instituted patient shadowing initiatives for physicians and nurses (Cleveland Clinic 2016), but we have not seen any evaluations of this program. However, we applaud these efforts and encourage other healthcare institutions to use this and our models to establish such programs for their staffs.

Chapter 6

The Leaflet Project

Contributions by Kilian Kelly

This chapter discusses a research project undertaken by the class, "Research Experience in Patient Provider Interaction" (chapter 3). The class incorporates a variety of research projects within the class. The initial research project in the first year of the class was an open-ended investigation of patient perspectives on what they did and did not understand about the Emergency Department (ED), their experiences, both positive and negative, and a comparison of those perspectives with those of the Emergency Medicine (EM) physicians. Based on the findings of the class—which focused on misunderstandings of what the ED could do and not do—the identity of the various personnel who treated them, and the time necessary for ED tests, the second class created and tested a leaflet designed to address these misunderstandings. Other organizations have attempted to create patient information leaflets in the past. However, this leaflet was based on data specifically generated from patient observation (patient shadowing) and qualitative interview data with the goal of being patient centric. After the creation of the initial leaflet, several students followed up on the project to continue the efforts to operationalize the use of the leaflets in the ED—a process that requires several administrative steps and approvals by multiple organization team members. Below is an overview of the background issues and current state of the project to date, which was coordinated by Kilian Kelly (an undergraduate anthropology student in the class who continued work on the project in the semesters after he completed the class; he has now completed a master's degree in anthropology). After a discussion of the issues involved in emergency room in general, we present a review of other published leaflets. This is followed by the presentation of the leaflet project that has been undertaken in the ED of Tampa General Hospital (TGH). This project is focused on representing actual patient informational needs within the leaflet. Through a review of past leaflets and extensive patient and key-stakeholder interviewing, a near-final product was produced that serves as the best representation of what a leaflet can accomplish when it is truly patient-centered.

BACKGROUND

The ED continues to be a widely used service in the United States, with over 145.6 million people seeking ED care in 2016 (CDC 2016). As these patients navigate the ED process, often they enter and exit without ever having a clear understanding of what the ED is designed to do or specifically how the ED functions. The lack of understanding ED processes and mismatches between patient expectations and ED realities often time leads to patients leaving the ED with more questions than they came in with initially—or, even worse, leaving without ever seeing a treatment provider. Patient experience measured using patient satisfaction surveys, such as the Press-Ganey Survey, are increasingly being tied to hospital and provider reimbursement. In addition, patients who leave without being seen represent a population of people that often returns to the ED even sicker, but who also represent uncaptured revenue for the hospital. In addition, the percent of patients who leave without being seen from the ED is a publicly reportable metric (hospitalcompare.gov). All these issues emphasize the importance of patients staying in the ED for evaluation and having a good experience of care while in the ED (Sonis et al. 2018).

A patient ED encounter involves interaction with numerous staff members who are not involved in the direct physician care team. Additional challenges in the ED include overcrowding, inadequate environmental hygiene, poor communication, unmet time management expectations, and minimized privacy (patients may need to be seen in hallways), all of which heavily influence the way the patient perceives their care (Sonis et al. 2018; Taylor and Benger 2004; Nairn et al. 2004). Patients usually do not have the medical knowledge to evaluate the overall care they receive and instead use environment proxies to make judgments about the quality of care they receive. Specifically, prior work has shown that even one unmet expectation in the ED (dirty chair, overcrowding, being evaluated in a non-private area) can create mistrust. One study found that increases in these proxy factors can also be linked to increases in patient complaints and lawsuits filed against the hospital, with the most pressing complaints being provider time spent with patient and notions of concern/courtesy toward patients (Stelfox et al. 2005). In contrast, increased patient satisfaction has been linked to increased compliance with treatment plans and better overall health outcomes (Sonis et al. 2018; Tamblyn et al. 2010). Often mismatches between patient visit expectations and physician goals lead to patient frustration. Furthermore, pain management has been cited by Body (2013) as a common area of patient-provider mismatch. Improvement in communication during the ED visit may help elucidate the scope of the ED and align provider-patient goals.

The current healthcare system is undergoing multiple reforms, but it has a deeply engrained non-patient-centered culture that will take years to correct. Present and future ED and hospital-wide changes should be patient centered and generated from data related specifically to patient needs, in line with lean processes which emphasize adding value to the patient experience.

But even with patient satisfaction surveys being distributed by hospitals, there is still little actual patient feedback used in new programming for institutions and providers to be immediately incorporated into exploratory interventions (Taylor and Benger, 2004; Sonis et al. 2018). There is a temporal gap and loss of information between nationally collected patient experience data, potential areas to focus on to locally improve patient experiences, and hospital interventions, including new patient-centric programs and materials that are distributed to patients.

Some institutions have distributed educational leaflets that attempt to answer the questions patients most often ask to improve patient satisfaction. These leaflets are most often distributed at registration or at other areas early in the patient care process. Nationally, however, patients may have low health literacy (between fourth and sixth grade reading level), and a common criticism of patient leaflets is that the reading level is too high or that the information contained is more advertisement than information of value to a patient during a care encounter. However, if patient-centered leaflets are created, they may be a tool that could reduce patient uncertainty, decrease the mismatch gap between patients and physicians, and reduce uncertainty about the overall ED experience. Previously distributed leaflets have not clearly addressed actual patient needs and may also not be accessible to the highly diverse populations that are served in most EDs.

REVIEW OF OTHER LEAFLETS

Educational patient leaflets are used in several EDs throughout the United States, Canada, and the United Kingdom. The methods utilized in the creation of these leaflets varied by location, thus leading to a wide range of final products that have been introduced to patients. Many of these other leaflets have inconsistencies in the extent to which the patient voice was considered during their development. Even in the case of leaflets which were meant to be made to include patient feedback for the improvement of the patient experience, it is not always clear if administrators have fully incorporated the information patients need most. Often, instead of a resource that can ease the process for patients, the leaflet can add to patient stress because of the inaccessibility of the information, even when it is in their hands.

The major components of leaflets that must be considered from the patient's perspective include the color palate, the reading level (whether the writing in the leaflet is at so high a reading level that the average patient cannot understand the material), and the overall wordiness of each page. We prefer to keep the reading level at about the fifth grade level to ensure health literacy. Reading level and overall look of a leaflet influence how approachable the leaflet is to a reader and how much of the patient's attention it can garner and hold. We evaluated other institution leaflets based on overall color and theme, reading level, and density of text, and created our own leaflet learning from these opportunities. We also directly integrated patient-generated information in order to create a patient-centric product.

Anderson Regional Medical Center in Mississippi created an educational leaflet in their ED (figure 6 1) that is not the strongest in terms of approachability and accessibility (Anderson Regional Medical Clinic). It is a two-page handout with a stock photo of a healthcare provider superimposed as the background of the first page. This background image makes the text a little difficult to read as it distorts the way the text both looks on the page and will be perceived by the reader. The entire first page is block text with practically no empty space. This is not inviting to a patient, as these large blocks of text seem cumbersome, even if the information is good. This background and text obscurity can be seen in figure6.1. Overall, the information on the first page is helpful, but it is at a high reading level and is not broken up with clip art or images. This may make it inaccessible to patients with less education and/or non-fluent English speakers. Others may not have the time or patience to read all the material, leading to this information being lost on these patients. The second page mainly focuses on food options, parking, and the pharmacy. This page is much stronger than the first one because not as much text is included. However, it is unclear if this page is meant for patients or for visitors, as the information on dining might be less relevant to the patient.

A well-designed leaflet should indicate which information is directly meant for patients and which information is intended for visitors. In addition, when outlining dining options, a leaflet should stress that all patients should first check with a healthcare team member whether they are cleared to eat, as many hospital procedures and medical conditions require a patient to not eat for a specific amount of time (often overnight before a morning test). This leaflet could be improved by reducing the wordiness on the first page, including more imagery, and reducing the size of the parking map so that there would be more space to spread out all the text on the first page.

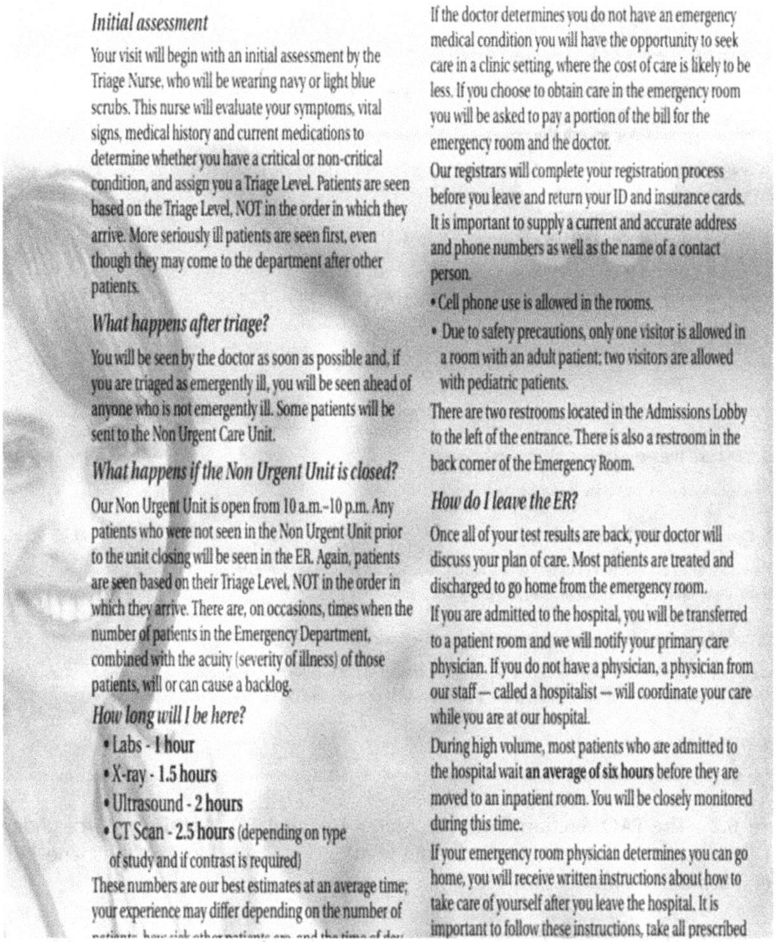

Initial assessment

Your visit will begin with an initial assessment by the Triage Nurse, who will be wearing navy or light blue scrubs. This nurse will evaluate your symptoms, vital signs, medical history and current medications to determine whether you have a critical or non-critical condition, and assign you a Triage Level. Patients are seen based on the Triage Level, NOT in the order in which they arrive. More seriously ill patients are seen first, even though they may come to the department after other patients.

What happens after triage?

You will be seen by the doctor as soon as possible and, if you are triaged as emergently ill, you will be seen ahead of anyone who is not emergently ill. Some patients will be sent to the Non Urgent Care Unit.

What happens if the Non Urgent Unit is closed?

Our Non Urgent Unit is open from 10 a.m.–10 p.m. Any patients who were not seen in the Non Urgent Unit prior to the unit closing will be seen in the ER. Again, patients are seen based on their Triage Level, NOT in the order in which they arrive. There are, on occasions, times when the number of patients in the Emergency Department, combined with the acuity (severity of illness) of those patients, will or can cause a backlog.

How long will I be here?

- Labs - **1 hour**
- X-ray - **1.5 hours**
- Ultrasound - **2 hours**
- CT Scan - **2.5 hours** (depending on type of study and if contrast is required)

These numbers are our best estimates at an average time; your experience may differ depending on the number of

If the doctor determines you do not have an emergency medical condition you will have the opportunity to seek care in a clinic setting, where the cost of care is likely to be less. If you choose to obtain care in the emergency room you will be asked to pay a portion of the bill for the emergency room and the doctor.

Our registrars will complete your registration process before you leave and return your ID and insurance cards. It is important to supply a current and accurate address and phone numbers as well as the name of a contact person.

- Cell phone use is allowed in the rooms.
- Due to safety precautions, only one visitor is allowed in a room with an adult patient; two visitors are allowed with pediatric patients.

There are two restrooms located in the Admissions Lobby to the left of the entrance. There is also a restroom in the back corner of the Emergency Room.

How do I leave the ER?

Once all of your test results are back, your doctor will discuss your plan of care. Most patients are treated and discharged to go home from the emergency room.

If you are admitted to the hospital, you will be transferred to a patient room and we will notify your primary care physician. If you do not have a physician, a physician from our staff – called a hospitalist – will coordinate your care while you are at our hospital.

During high volume, most patients who are admitted to the hospital wait **an average of six hours** before they are moved to an inpatient room. You will be closely monitored during this time.

If your emergency room physician determines you can go home, you will receive written instructions about how to take care of yourself after you leave the hospital. It is important to follow these instructions, take all prescribed

Figure 6.1 "Welcome to the Emergency Department." *Source*: The Anderson Regional Medical Clinic Anderson Regional Medical Center.

Mater Hospital Brisbane did not have a physical leaflet available, but we did identify a patient web link with similar information formatted in the style of a leaflet (figure 6.2) (Mater Hospital Brisbane 2011). The website displays a general lack of images and color besides the header. The only way the large amount of text is broken up is by headers that are in slightly larger font size and in blue instead of black text. The reading level of this page is lower, making it far more accessible to more patients, though it is unclear if this information is widely distributed or if patients must go out of their way to find it. If it is the latter, then there is a major disparity in who can access this, as it assumes that all patients will have stable internet access and know

FAQs

1. What happens if I get worse while I am waiting?

Please notify the Triage Nurse if your condition has changed or if your pain worsens.

2. Will it cost anything to visit the Emergency Department?

Australian citizens receive free care. Some services are bulk-billed to Medicare. Non-Australian citizens may be charged if they are not from countries with reciprocal arrangements with Australia.

3. What if I don't understand what I am meant to do?

Please ask questions of our staff if you do not understand what is happening. Ask for a written discharge plan if you think it will help with your health care. We can also send a letter to your GP.

4. Can I smoke?

Mater has a strict NO SMOKING policy in all of its buildings.

5. Can I use the vending machines, eat or drink?

Please consult with the Triage Nurse before eating and drinking.

6. Can I use my mobile phone?

Please consider the comfort of others in the Waiting Room. Out of courtesy for staff and other patients, please refrain from use of mobile phones within the Emergency Department.

7. Can I have friends or relatives in the Department with me?

We understand the importance of having the support of friends and relatives. We will do our best to accommodate your needs. Please understand that we may place a restriction for some health care procedures or if space is limited.

8. Where can I park?

The space outside the Emergency Department is for drop-off and pick-up only. Mater Health Services provide car

Figure 6.2 The FAQ Section from the Mater Hospital ED Website. *Source*: Adapted from "Welcome to the Emergency Department" from Mater Hospital Brisbane (2011). Mater Hospital Brisbane.

where to look for the information. It also includes a FAQ section at the end, which is both informative and concise. This is the strongest section of this website (figure 6.2), as it does not overwhelm readers with large blocks of text and is informative. The best improvement would be to convert this into a handout that can be given to patients so that they do not have to search for the information themselves.

St. Thomas Elgin General Hospital in Ontario distributes a flow chart that details the patient flow through the ED (STEGH) (figure 6.3). This is an engaging way to present the information because it breaks up the text by using boxes and gives a direct path of progression. This flow chart is shown below in figure 6.3. It is just one page, so it does not overwhelm patients with a large amount of material to read while they are waiting. Despite this, however, the flow chart is bland and unappealing. There is no color or images to attract the eye. The flow chart provides a good layout of expected throughput

WELCOME TO THE EMERGENCY DEPARTMENT
UPON ARRIVAL
You will be assessed bv a Triaoe Nurse to ensure the most serious cases are treated first
NEXT....REGISTRATION
A Registration Clerk will ask some questions and place a patient identification band on your
TO WAITING ROOM
Some patients may be called into a treatment room before you, even if they arrived after you
We make every attempt to keep your waiting time as short as possible
If you are concerned at any time while waiting or you feel your condition has changed, please speak to the triage nurse
Most serious injury or condition among all patients?
TO TREATMENT ROOM
A nurse will evaluate your condition and ask you about your medical history, current medications and allergies
A physician or resident will perform an examination and ask more questions
Tests or other procedures may be ordered
Test results and diagnostic procedures can take time to be completed and for the results to be available
A decision will be made to either send you home or admit you to hospital
If you are going home, discharge instructions will be given to you by the physician or nurse and any other information regarding prescriptions, follow-up tests, or appointments will be provided at this time.

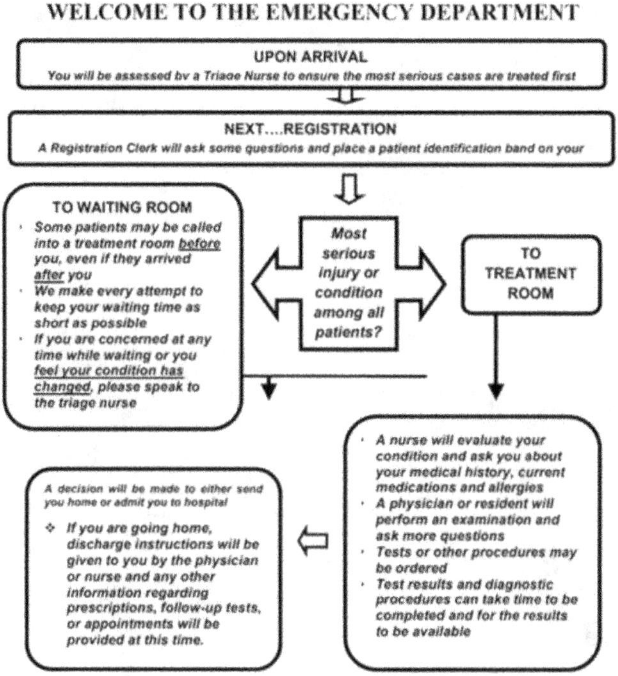

Figure 6.3 Adapted from "Welcome to the Emergency Department" from the STEGH.
Source: STEGH.

as patients move through the ED but does not do anything to address other expectations patients may have about their care. The diagram does not describe wait times for treatments or tests. Healthcare team member roles are not delineated. The leaflet leaves the reader without clear understanding of ED process, or why the flow occurs in the manner outlined on the diagram. If a leaflet is not going to adequately inform or educate patients, there doesn't seem to be a purpose in providing that leaflet to patients, as it will just cause more confusion.

The Gifford Medical Center in Vermont produced a trifold leaflet that covered many important topics for ED patients, including arrival and admission, waiting, comfort, and discharge (figure 6.4). The overall leaflet is bland in color, utilizing mostly a greyscale, but the addition of green accents for the headers and other details is appealing. In terms of content, the amount of text used is rather overwhelming, the font size is small, and the reading level is quite high. This color scale and wordiness is represented in the portion of the leaflet shown below in figure 6.4. This is not conducive to patient utilization of this leaflet, as it is not approachable and not engaging. There are not any images to help break up the text and even the section titles are lengthy and *"a crisis . . ."*

Managing pain

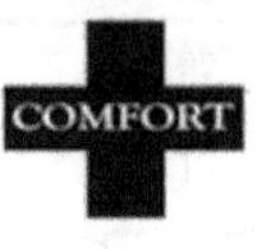

To help you understand what you can expect from your visit to Gifford's Emergency Department, a description of the hospital's Pain Management Guidelines follows.

1) Your Emergency Department provider will objectively assess your pain and, depending on your type of injury, will only prescribe narcotic pain medicine if deemed appropriate.

2) Your Emergency Department provider may not fill a specific pain management request despite what has been provided to you in the past.

3) Patients visiting from out of the area or who have no local health care provider will not be given a prescription for a controlled substance for a chronic pain condition.

4) Prescriptions for controlled or narcotic medicines will be limited to one per month or three per year for patients whose pain cannot be discerned by the Emergency Department provider, such as back or dental pain.

5) Patients who have a pain treatment plan established with their primary care provider will not be given refills for controlled or narcotic medicines. Rather, you will be referred back to your primary health care provider for the prescription.

6) No prescriptions for longacting narcotics will be given except in unique circumstances, such as for cancer pain.

7) Patients with a known history of drug abuse or criminal behavior related to drugs will not be given a prescription for narcotics from an Emergency Department provider.

Continuing your care after discharge

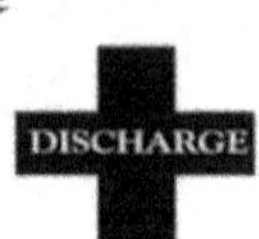

Patients should arrange for care or follow-up appointments as directed in their Emergency Department discharge instructions.

Gifford strongly recommends that you develop a relationship with a primary care provider to maintain continuity of your care. By choosing a personal provider from the Gifford community, you can build a trusted relationship with a provider who has a thorough knowledge of your medical history and needs. For a copy of the Gifford Provider Directory, call (802) 728-2284 or visit Registration.

What is HCAHPS?

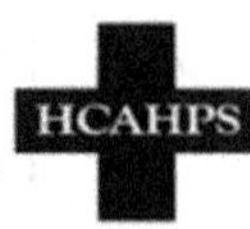

HCAHPS is a mandated standardized survey of patients' perspectives of hospital care. HCAHPS *(Hospital Consumer Assessment of Healthcare Providers and Systems)* measures patients' perceptions of their hospital experience through a series of 27 questions. The survey is mailed to patients between 48 hours and six weeks after discharge. When you receive a survey, please note that survey questions refer to your "Doctor," which you should interpret as **your provider in the hospital,** not your primary care physician. Your provider will be a hospitalist, which may include physicians and physician assistants.

Figure 6.4 Adapted from "Welcome to the Emergency Department" from the Gifford Medical Center. *Source*: Gifford Medical Center.

overly verbose. It seems to have been written by providers who may have thought they were answering questions they anticipated their patient might have during the encounter. But, in fact, they were just conveying the issues they saw, using their own vernacular. The information is appropriate but is not actually helpful because it is not written in a way that can be used by patients who may have low health literacy. This is an excellent example of a leaflet that on the surface was created to be for patients but misses the opportunity to create a patient-centric literature. This leaflet is designed more for medical professionals more than for patients who will be reading the material. To improve on this leaflet, the amount of text and the reading level both need to be drastically lowered. The most important points in the leaflet should be better emphasized and excess material could be removed. There should also be more images included to break up the text and increase readability.

England has a National Healthcare System (NHS), and some of the pressures on patient experience are different than in the United States. Nonetheless, optimal patient experience remains an important component in

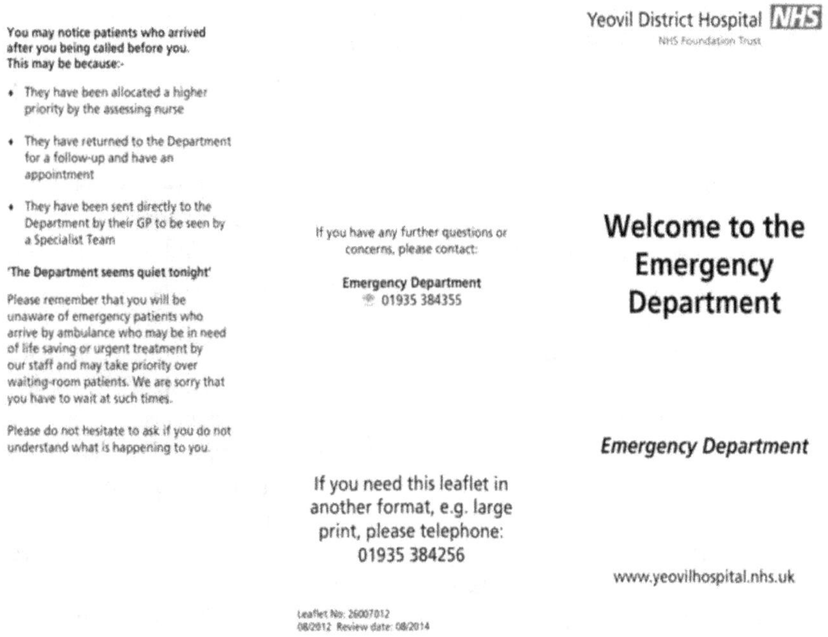

You may notice patients who arrived after you being called before you. This may be because:-

- They have been allocated a higher priority by the assessing nurse
- They have returned to the Department for a follow-up and have an appointment
- They have been sent directly to the Department by their GP to be seen by a Specialist Team

'The Department seems quiet tonight'

Please remember that you will be unaware of emergency patients who arrive by ambulance who may be in need of life saving or urgent treatment by our staff and may take priority over waiting-room patients. We are sorry that you have to wait at such times.

Please do not hesitate to ask if you do not understand what is happening to you.

If you have any further questions or concerns, please contact:

Emergency Department
01935 384355

If you need this leaflet in another format, e.g. large print, please telephone: 01935 384256

Leaflet No: 26007012
08/2012 Review date: 08/2014

Yeovil District Hospital NHS
NHS Foundation Trust

Welcome to the Emergency Department

Emergency Department

www.yeovilhospital.nhs.uk

Figure 6.5 Adapted from "Welcome to the Emergency Department" from the Yeovil Hospital (2014). *Source*: Yeovil Hospital.

building trust and following through with care plans. Yeovil District Hospital in Somerset, England, has a trifold leaflet that is distributed to patient in the ED (figure 6.5) (Yeovil District Hospital 2014). Overall, this leaflet appears bland and unappealing. The product manages to be simultaneously overly wordy but also has excess empty white space. It looks like the use of space was not well planned, and there was a considerable amount of wasted space. These large white spaces and blocks of text can be seen in figure 6.5. The leaflet does not appear to have undergone an extensive amount of planning prior to creation. There is no color used outside of colors for the text denoting the levels of urgency for different levels of inpatient cases, and there are no images. There are large white spaces where images could easily have been inserted, but instead, they were just left empty. The information itself is also sparse, and a lot of useful information for patients is not included.

Our research, including observations in the ED waiting room, has consistently demonstrated that patients become frustrated when they recognize that regular American cultural rules of turn taking do not apply as patients are seen in order of severity (determined by triage nurse), not in order of arrival. In addition, throughput facilitation and resource utilization also may guide how quickly a patient is seen and discharged or admitted. In other words, a patient that needs a quick medication refill or staple removal might be placed directly in front of a physician or other provider and quickly discharged from the ED while a patient that requires a thorough examination, more history, and diagnostic imaging might be sent back to the waiting room after triage.

The NHS leaflet does have an area that covers this topic, as well as the general expected patient flow in the ED. However, that information is superficial. The reading level is more appropriate for the ED patient. Overall, to improve on this leaflet, the text and blank space ratio should be balanced out with images, and the actual text should also be enhanced to address the shortcomings we have addressed.

The Exeter Hospital ED in New Hampshire produced a one-page handout that included a very superficial, though dense, overview of ED patient throughput (Exeter Hospital 2014; figure 6.6). This handout uses poor color choice and the leaflet appears dreary. The leaflet is not likely to be read completely or in detail by a patient. The pale blue with black text does not engage the reader. The Exeter ED handout is shown below in figure 6.6. There is too much text and minimal imagery to reduce the text blocks. The reading level is also high, above the average ED patient health literacy level.

Information regarding the ED "Physician First" process appears first and indicates that the physicians are at the front lines of the treatment process

Exeter Hospital Emergency Department Now Offers *PhysicianFirst*

Our new *PhysicianFirst* triage process, introduced by EMP for peak volume times, means that you are evaluated by a physician when you first come into the Emergency Department (ED). The physician and nurse make a rapid assessment of your needs while you are being checked in. They can then order blood tests and medications, start an IV, and determine the next steps before you are even brought back to an ED patient room. This new process ensures you receive care sooner and decreases wait times.

What Happens After Triage?

After you have been assessed, you may be discharged to go home or brought to a room in the ED.

When Will I Go to a Room?

Patients are assigned ED rooms based on the severity of their illness or injury. More critical patients are seen first, whether they walk in or arrive by ambulance. Triage helps to determine each patient's need.

What Happens Next?

In the ED room, you may have tests such as blood work or X-Rays. You will then be treated by the physicians, physician assistants and nurses. Depending on your condition, you will then be discharged or admitted to a room in the hospital for further testing or care.

Being Discharged

When you are discharged, you will be given instructions for any follow up care that is needed. Be sure to ask any final questions you may have. It is important to follow up with your primary care provider as directed. **If you don't have a primary care provider, please call our Information & Referral Center at 603-580-6668 and our staff will help you find a provider who meets your personal needs.**

Your Feedback is Important

Most patients will be sent a survey about your care after you return home. We take your feedback seriously, so please take a moment to fill out the survey. If you have a specific praise or concern, you can call our patient relations coordinator at 603-580-6913. **Thank you for choosing the Exeter Hospital Emergency Department.**
Your care is our priority.

Figure 6.6 Adapted from "Welcome to Exeter Hospital Emergency Department" from Exeter Hospital (2014). *Source*: Exeter Hospital.

from start to finish. The high reading level and style of the writing ("peak volume times," "triage process") suggest that this text may have been written by the physicians themselves, half advertisement, and half patient information. We felt that the Exeter ED handout represented an example of what not to do given the overall appearance, high reading level, and writing style likely leading to a low retention rate of the information and low success of the leaflet in helping close the gap between patient and physician/institution expectations during the ED visit.

New South Wales (NSW) Government Health has released a trifold leaflet that is both engaging and informative (figure 6.7) (NSW 2011). The color blocks with the bright yellow, red, white, and black are exciting and keep the reader moving through the presented information. The NSW leaflet has the best color palette of any of the previously discussed examples. Unfortunately, the NSW does still suffer from an overall lack of images, but the creator's use of colors and different shapes in the text boxes at least breaks up some of the text. The text itself is still quite dense, with a high reading level surpassing

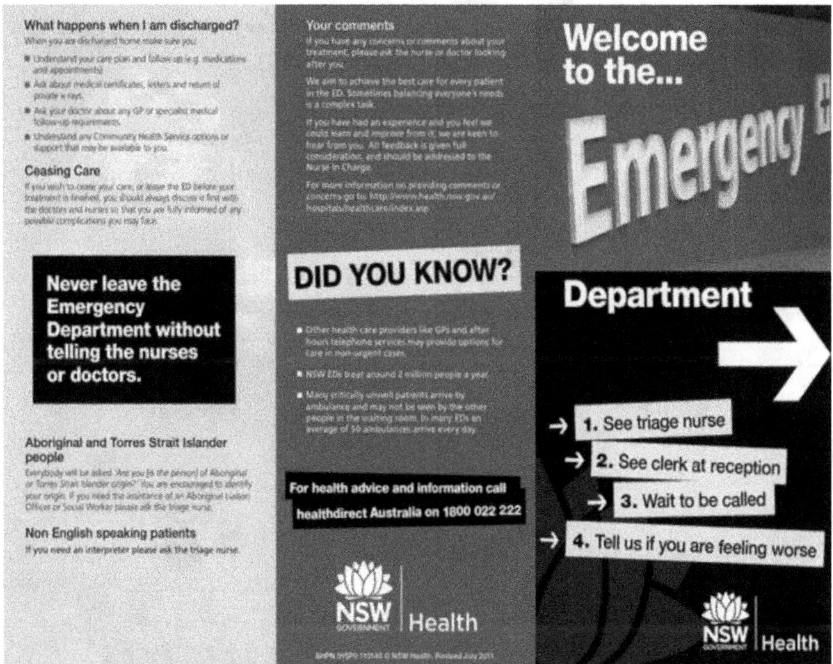

Figure 6.7 Exemplifies the diverse and engaging color palette used by the NSW. The use of warm tones and color blocking makes it easier to read and less dreary to look at as a reader. Though It Does Also Highlight the Still Dense Use of Text with a Decently High Reading Level. Adapted from "Welcome to the . . . Emergency Department" from NSW Government Health (2011). *Source*: NSW Government Health.

the health literacy level of most ED patients. The leaflet makes use of blocks of text as do many of the other discussed leaflets, but the designers counterbalanced some of the text blocks with the use of the text boxes and color. This leaflet is an excellent example of how engaging colors and images can make an otherwise text-based leaflet far more approachable and inviting to readers. The leaflet does a good job of touching on a wide range of topics that are of interest to patients, such as the trajectory of care, visitor information, and triage, wait times. The reading level and amount of text should be reduced and replaced with images.

The Children's Hospital of Eastern Ontario has one of the best leaflets reviewed. The leaflet is exciting to look at and the information is helpful (figure 6.8) (CHEO 2012). The CHEO leaflet minimizes the use of large text blocks. Bright and engaging colors are used along with clip art with images to create shorter sections of text. The leaflet designers use electric green and blue as accent colors which make the leaflet more dynamic and exciting. The

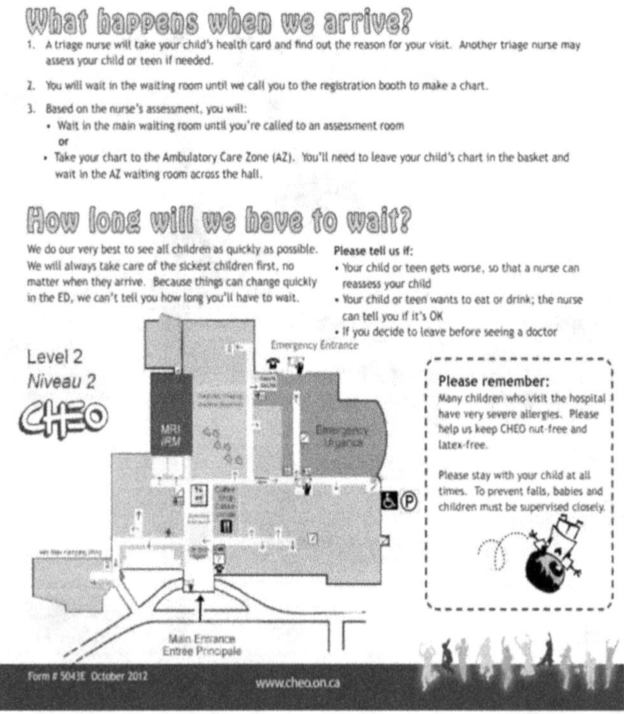

Figure 6.8 A Small Section of the CHEO Leaflet. This image shows some of the bright colors and images used throughout the leaflet that make it engaging and more readable as it is not bogged down with large chunks of text. Adapted from "Welcome to our Emergency Department (ED)" from CHEO (2012). *Source*: CHEO.

text is also broken up with bullet points and small images that are relevant and engaging. The reading level is also far more on par with what would be most accessible to a wide variety of patients. The leaflet creators avoided complex terms that are not useful or necessary. There is little here that needs improvement; however, adding more images would further break up the text.

In our opinion, the UC Davis Medical Center produced the best leaflet that we reviewed. The UC Davis leaflet covered the widest range of the patient experience in a way that is accessible and engaging (figure 6.9) (UC Davis). We did not observe the same critical problems of the other leaflets in the UC Davis leaflet. The UC Davis leaflet is colorful and images were included on every page. The text is kept to a minimum, and the reading level is a much lower level than other comparable leaflets.

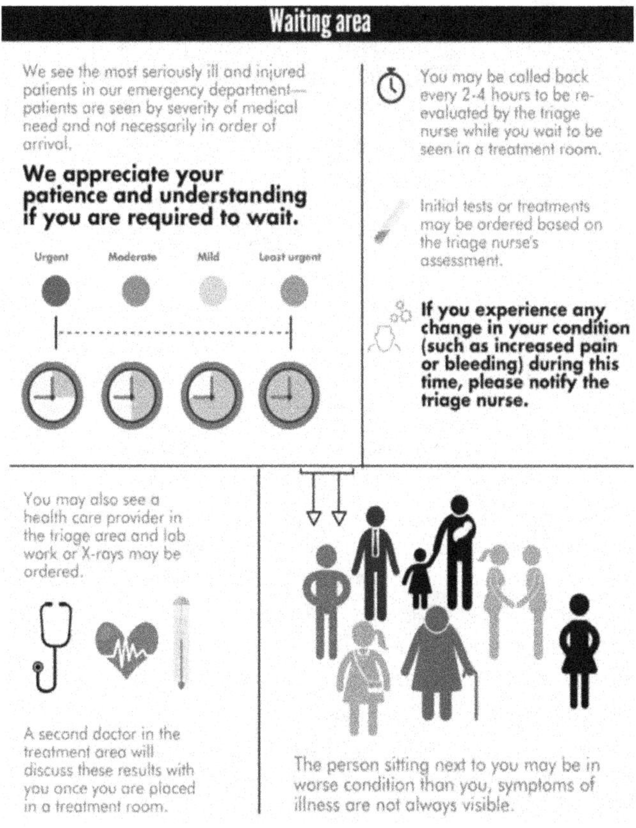

Figure 6.9 One Portion of the UC Davis leaflet where it discusses wait time. It highlights both the excellent use of language but also the adept use of imagery and color to boost engagement and accessibility. Adapted from "Welcome to the UC Davis Medical Center Emergency Department" from UC Davis. *Source*: UC Davis Health.

The UC Davis leaflet illustrates an exemplar of how to convey important wait time information while explaining the nonnormative style of turn taking that occurs in an ED waiting room to explain the order patients will be seen (figure 6.9 shows this section). The use of imagery and the explanations of severity as the deciding factor in determining the order patients are seen the best we have seen among all of the leaflets we reviewed. We feel that conveying the reason for wait times and for a deviation from standard turn taking based on severity are key aspects of a successful ED leaflet.

Our review of previously created leaflets indicates that other institutions have attempted to relay important information to patients and to address the expectation mismatch, potentially improving the patient experience of care. However, when we considered gaps between an ideal leaflet and an available leaflet, this review of other leaflets served as an important first step to emphasize key opportunities in our leaflet design. Our goal was to create a TGH ED leaflet based directly on observations, interviews, and data gathered from TGH ED patients and present that information back to patients, addressing their concerns and questions in a way that is both accessible and able to be widely understood regardless of health literacy level.

METHODS

To begin the creation of a new leaflet, the class conducted qualitative research about patient informational needs. The class members conducted 237 total hours of participant observation at various points in the ED. Areas of observation included the registration desk, triage pivot rooms—a location where patients are "pivoted" between more sick (or requiring a bed during entire ED stay) and not as sick (potentially able to stay moving throughout the ED during the encounter)—patient waiting areas, pods (areas of the ED where physicians, nurses, and other support staff work in divided areas to break up the ED census into more manageable units), patient rooms, and the physician desks. Participant observation was carried out to gain a better understanding of the discrete flow through the ED and to experience the ED throughput process from the patient lens at each step.

Following participant observation, students in the course then participated in physician and patient shadowing. Shadowing experiences (also described in more detail in chapter 3) included 64 hours shadowing physicians and 128 hours shadowing patients across all students.

The ED field site is an urban Level 1 trauma and tertiary care center associated with a medical school. The physicians work across multiple "pods" in order to better organize a 62-bed ED. Pod 1 is the pediatric pod, and pod 2 is where patients that are admitted and waiting for a bed in the hospital are cohorted for more efficient "boarding" (the healthcare term that describes patients who are admitted and waiting for placement in the hospital). Pods 3, 4, and 5 are all 10-bed adult patient pods which also accommodate 2 to 4 hallway beds in each area. There is also an eight-bed trauma bay. Students spent time in Pods 3, 4, and 5 and the trauma bay. One attending physician (supervising doctor that has completed residency training) oversees each pod and the group of attending physicians split duties in the trauma bay.

Students in the course were assigned to a pod and attending physician to conduct physician shadowing. In each pod, the attending physician usually had one to two assigned residents and a medical student. The students each followed the attending physician, unless the attending physician requested that the student also spend time shadowing the resident. The student shadowed each patient encounter and interaction that took place over a four-hour period as well as any other staff interactions or administrative tasks to get a better understanding of ED time from the physician perspective.

During patient shadowing (described more in chapter 3), students were paired with a patient who had just been placed either in a hallway bed or in a room, early in the ED course. The student then sat with the patient, following the patient to all diagnostic tests, and witnessing all staff and physician interactions, until the patient reached a disposition (discharge from the ED or admission to the hospital). Patient shadowing allowed the students to see and feel exactly how the process felt when they were in the position of the patient vis-à-vis the physician. This also allowed students to gain a much clearer view of what the patients were feeling while they moved through the process, and what questions they were asking most frequently during their ED course.

Once the shadowing was completed, each student created their own version of a leaflet that each thought best represented what they had observed while conducting the participant observation and shadowing activities. The students then returned to the waiting room and each showed their leaflet to a selection of patients to get direct patient feedback on what they liked and did not like. The students met again and discussed the patient feedback and their peer comments. This led to the development of 15 different leaflets that were compared and discussed in a classroom setting, looking for common themes or unique and important areas for concentration. Through this process, students created a single leaflet utilizing the feedback and points of emphasis that were raised through class discussion, participant observation, shadowing, and leaflet sharing. This new leaflet was then retested in the waiting room and more revisions were made again based on patient feedback.

Once the final draft compiled version of that leaflet was completed, over a thousand copies of the leaflet were printed, based on ED volume, to create a case control study. Our original design was to randomize weeks in the remaining part of the semester to be "leaflet weeks" and other weeks to be "non-leaflet" weeks creating our case and control samples. Students then conducted semi-structured interviews with patients who were being discharged from the ED. This occurred over several weeks, where some weeks the leaflets were being distributed to every patient who came through registration and other weeks where the leaflet was not distributed. This allowed the students to observe whether the patients were more satisfied with their care and better understood the ED when they had or did not have the leaflet. Patients in both groups were asked about their general experience in the ED, wait times, what was good about their visit, what was bad, and their general understanding of ED operations and throughput. Patients who were interviewed when the leaflet was in circulation were also asked about the leaflet, if they read it, if they found it helpful, what parts of it were the most successful, what parts needed to be changed, and if there was anything they felt was missing from it.

The project, like most research and Quality Improvement (QI) efforts taking place in the field, was not without challenges. Midway through data collection, the hospital marketing team became aware of the project. They took the class leaflet out of circulation. To gain approval for the leaflet to reenter circulation, we agreed to a few changes requested by the marketing team so that the leaflet fit better with their desired aesthetic for hospital educational materials. Interestingly, one of the direct quotes from the marketing team was: "We can't have material at this low of a reading level being distributed with our logo on it—that reflects poorly on us, like we don't have a grasp of writing and grammar."

This quote and perspective emphasize the challenge of moving healthcare from a physician- and organization-centered activity to one that places patient needs front and center.

After the marketing team approved the release of the modified leaflet, there were now two different leaflets being examined during the semester-long study period. The first leaflet was, we feel, more patient focused while the second was modified to be more hospital focused. Students compiled all leaflet data, stratified by each leaflet, compared patient feedback for non-leaflet and leaflet weeks, and then presented to hospital stakeholders as a group oral presentation led by the students.

Hospital stakeholders were tentatively supportive of a patient-centered leaflet, but each felt strongly that their area of supervision and responsibility should be represented appropriately and in line with the larger hospital mission, vision, and strategies. We felt that these concerns were likely not as important to the patients for whom the leaflet was created, but also recognized the administrative challenges of a large healthcare organization, especially in terms of releasing collateral material and publications displaying the institution logo. Thus, we agreed to work with individual stakeholders to get their buy-in and open the leaflet for modifications that would not detract from the overall goal of being patient-centered, not organization centric.

Individual key-stakeholder interviews began with several people in various departments in the hospital. We felt strongly that the leaflet should become a permanent ED fixture and thus would have to move through approval by a chain of departments and people.

The project had been mostly student run up to this point; however, course faculty (JWW and RDB) reached out to the Chief Operating Officer (COO) of the hospital who was a former ED nurse with a solid understanding of patient-physician expectation mismatches and the important need to improve the patient experience. The director of Patient Experience also attended this meeting and course faculty received strong support to move the project to key hospital leaders, opening the door for an undergraduate honors student to continue work on the project as part of their honors thesis (Kilian Kelly). Key stakeholders who were interviewed included the director of the marketing, the nursing director of the ED, and the education director for the ED. Additional interviews also took place between Kilian Kelly and the director of Patient Experience. These interviews were vital in finding a fair balance between the desired focus on patient experience and perspective, and the hospital's need for consistent branding and aesthetics. Some of the major information that was consistent across these key-stakeholder interviews was the need for consistency in reading level and amount of text. Fortunately, we did reach agreement that it was appropriate to keep the reading level low, around that of the fourth grade. There was also a consensus to reduce the overall amount of text so that the leaflet would not appear tedious or intimidating to patients. All this information was compiled with all the patient interview data to create a final product that both reflected the needs of the patient and maintained the image and voice of the hospital. This was then reintroduced to ED via registration and semi-structured interviews were again conducted with the patients with the newest edition of the leaflet. That data was compared to the data collected previously on the other two versions of the leaflet.

RESULTS

Initial class qualitative data that were used in the development of the class leaflet included field notes from the patient shadowing experiences undertaken by students. These were coded and analyzed, revealing important themes that were incorporated into the educational leaflet. Healthcare team and provider communication, as well as communication regarding wait times, were a consistent theme across student shadowing experiences that had a large impact on the overall patient experience. Data from student observations demonstrated that patients often misunderstood medical terminology and that staff often overestimated the medical knowledge and vocabulary of their patients. Medical jargon and advanced healthcare language were not used exclusively by physicians. Other members of the healthcare team, including nurses, paramedics, and patient care technicians, also use similar terminology that was above the health literacy level of the patient population. Our data demonstrate that patients recognized when advanced language was being used that they did not fully understand, but instead of demanding explanation or a change in communication style, patients instead became upset and had a worse overall experience. In addition, communication gaps led many patients to question the care they received, as they did not understand what was happening. One of the students noted, "The patient had an 8th-9th grade reading level and the resident had asked questions about the patient's baseline creatinine level . . . I got to see the patient's reaction: scared, restless."

Student observations indicated patients' fear and discomfort when being confronted with medical jargon used by the healthcare team without explanation. Diagnoses were sometimes lost in the discourse, with patients being unaware of their diagnosis until they read it in their discharge paperwork (which is also challenging to understand secondary to high use of medical terms and an advanced reading level).

One patient even stated, "I thought talking to her [the physician] would give me some clarity, but it just made me more confused."

Our data from student observations and shadowing also highlight differences in the way patients and physicians experience the ED. Patients and healthcare staff have different definitions of "emergency." In addition, and perhaps most striking, the passage of time differs greatly between patients and physicians—a phenomenon noted by multiple students over the years we have been teaching the course.

This issue has been addressed by the medical community. The "prudent layperson standard" was enacted to protect the understood differences between what physicians and patients consider to be an emergency. In the state of Washington, to try and curb Medicaid and other insurance program payments, numerous attempts have been made to allow payers to only reimburse ED visits if the diagnosis was an emergent diagnosis. Instead, patient rights groups and EM physicians have worked to ensure that if a patient comes to the ED with that another "prudent layperson" might also think could represent an emergency, that should be enough to justify an ED encounter and payment for those services. For example, if an overweight 55-year-old male smoker with high cholesterol presents to the ED with chest pressure only to find his symptoms are from gastric reflux (GERD), that patient with those risk factors made a reasonable choice to seek care in an ED as that cluster of symptoms might have represented a myocardial infarct (heart attack).

ED physicians often communicated to the public that if you are having any symptoms that are not normal for you and you feel they are emergent, that should be enough to trigger an ED visit. From the payer, physician, patient, and hospital perspectives, the concept of what an emergency is remains important. From a patient experience perspective, physicians and healthcare staff must remember that they observe the same or similar cases multiple times every day. Thus, the standard of what constitutes emergency may shift within the setting of an ED where all the present population may all feel they have an emergency. The bar is raised both consciously and subconsciously as staff sort patients into emergent but not life-threatening right now to a more urgent category of patients with a current life-threatening condition. This leads to a disconnect between what the patient is feeling and experiencing and how the physician responds, impacting the patient's perception of care and their overall patient experience.

One of our students noted after a patient interview that "the patient believes anything that damages his/her daily routine or prevents him/her from working is considered an emergency. The physicians associate 'emergency' with life threatening conditions."

Negative patient experiences often are related to this designation of a non-emergency. Or put another way, physicians spend a lot of upfront time and investment with a patient, focusing on a thorough initial medical screening exam (MSE) and history. Often, an experienced physician will know right then if a patient has a definitive emergency. Other times, some patients may still have a possible emergency while still other patients may clearly not actually have an emergency or a feared diagnosis. Given the cadence of the ED, the emphasis on emergent disease states, and the time demands on staff and physicians, it becomes difficult to spend more time with patients after determining they do not have an emergency—which is why patient care pathways must be created for new ways of managing illness (e.g., opioid use disorder pathway). The work by Kleinman et al. (1978) remains relevant in this context.

To deliver a positive patient experience, physicians must be able to navigate between a non-emergent disease state and an ongoing illness, or present suffering of the patient as they explain next steps, other explanatory models, and why the feared disease is not actually present. In other words, EM physicians spend a great deal of time on the front end of the patient encounter but, for the non-emergent patient, a balance of more time on the back end better explaining the illness, next steps, and a discharge plan might be critical steps to improve patient satisfaction scores across lower severity ED patients. When the disease (determined to not be emergent) and the illness (still presenting as suffering by the patient) are disconnected, the patient is left feeling unsatisfied with their care and their experience in the

ED because they do not feel as if they were taken seriously by the healthcare team.

Almost every class we have taught has had students who commented on the vast difference in how time is experienced as a physician compared to a patient. Hours fly by when shadowing the physician as the team rushes around to see multiple patients and points along each patient care continuum are at different stages at any given time. Patient shadowing, on the other hand, revealed the slow boredom of sitting in one room waiting for sporadic encounters and bits of information being delivered by healthcare staff often without clear expectations of how long would pass before the next test, encounter, or completion of the ED visit.

Physicians are always moving, always doing something—they see patients, record their notes, and consult with the healthcare team; four hours spent shadowing a physician flies by in the blink of an eye, as there is little time when there is nothing happening (although to a patient staring out of an ED room, seeing physicians typing on computers and talking to other team members does not always convey this busy urgency of an ED shift). Patients experience time much more slowly. While sitting in the patient room, or sitting in the hallway, time drags. The prospect of progress or discharge seems so far off because, unlike for the physicians, for the patients, there is nothing to do. Patients have difficulty relaxing even with cable television and free wireless (although TV is harder to come by when patients are placed in the hallway) secondary to the state of waiting itself. There is also little understanding of the experiences of the other. Patients do not see all the physicians have to do over the course of their shift; they only see them when they are in the room, which often is less than two minutes each instance. Conversely, the physicians are moving too quickly to understand how stagnant things feel for the patients. This is further exacerbated by poor communication between the physicians and the patients. Time moves so quickly for the physicians that regular updates are not often provided to the patients regarding progress in their care.

After taking part in both the patient and physician shadowing, one of the students noted, "Physicians are busy and have multiple patients to deal with. For a patient, their perspective of what the physicians are doing is sitting around their desks, talking among themselves."

ED patients consistently have expressed confusion surrounding how the ED functions, staff roles, throughput, and processes, as well as abilities and scope of ED visits. This confusion was also a consistent theme among student observations, shadowing experiences, and interviews. Many patients were unclear about the way the ED is meant to run and why things happen in the way they do, leading to expectation mismatches that could not be overcome. One student noted that a particular patient "assumed everyone in the hospital was a doctor, which was very far from the truth. He called everyone doctor, no matter who they were."

Hospital staff do wear different color scrubs and identification badges stating roles such as patient care technician, registered nurse, paramedic, radiology technician, respiratory therapist, case manager, social worker, resident physician, attending physician, and pharmacist but many patients were unsure how to differentiate the scrub colors or what the specific identified roles meant in terms of their own ED experience. Patients were unsure what types of questions to ask each staff member. In addition, the overall abilities and role of the ED as an institution were unclear to patients. Patients were unsure what closure of their visit would look like and what the possible options were at disposition (patient would likely be discharged with follow-up, placed in an observation unit, admitted to another team of physicians and staff for further management, or taken more urgently for an operation or procedure). Lack of role and organizational knowledge led to more mismatched expectations as patients often expressed that they simply expected to come in, see a doctor, and have all their problems identified with a solution. Patients frequently underestimated the number of people they would meet over the course of their ED encounter and had little understanding regarding the scope of each staff member. Patients have an expectation for comprehensive care management in the ED.

The patient expectation of the ED encounter and the 24/7 nature of the discipline has frustrated policy makers in attempts to decrease healthcare spending by minimizing ED visits. Multiple efforts to decrease ED utilization, controversially seen as an expensive waste of healthcare dollars (even though EDs care for over 65% of unscheduled visits at less than 5% of all healthcare spending, ACEP 2015), have failed, with ED visits continuing to rise even as health insurance coverage has increased under the Affordable Care Act in the United States (Singer et al. 2019). A combination of convenience, patient cost, accessibility, and federal law requiring less upfront payment, as well as the availability of well-trained board-certified EM physicians and specialists has continued to drive patients to the ED. Perhaps ED encounters should be reimagined as unscheduled visits, allowing for upfront and intentional design and focus toward meeting that demand (Pines et al. 2016). Patients seek care in EDs after work, before work, on weekends and can get care often months sooner than what they would experience waiting for a primary care appointment.

Urban departments are often on major bus lines or in walking distance of population centers, creating easier accessibility for patients. The availability of laboratory services, imaging, and other diagnostic testing also allows patients to complete an encounter at one location, perhaps with one co-pay, instead of needing transportation all over town to visit multiple vendors. The

Emergency Medicine Treatment and Labor Act (EMTALA) also requires that every patient receive a MSE to rule out an emergent medical condition, prior to collection of payment (EMTALA, CMS Website), removing some financial barriers for the delivery of at least emergent or urgent care in the ED setting (urgent care centers are not subject to this federal law and, thus, require upfront payment). As we reimagine a patient-centered healthcare system, how can EDs and hospital systems function 24/7 to meet patient expectations in financially sustainable ways since this model of one-stop, anytime, care is clearly part of the patient's expectation?

The themes outlined here were central concerns that emerged in the class data and thus were addressed in the creation of the class leaflet. A focus on reading level, delivery of material, and tangible content was all important and emphasized. The initial leaflet that was created is shown below in figures 6.10 and 6.11. Once distributed, this leaflet version received positive patient feedback. Two hundred and eleven interviews were conducted in the ED, with leaflets being distributed on alternating weeks. Demographic breakdowns for the patients interviewed can be seen below in tables 6.1 and 6.2.

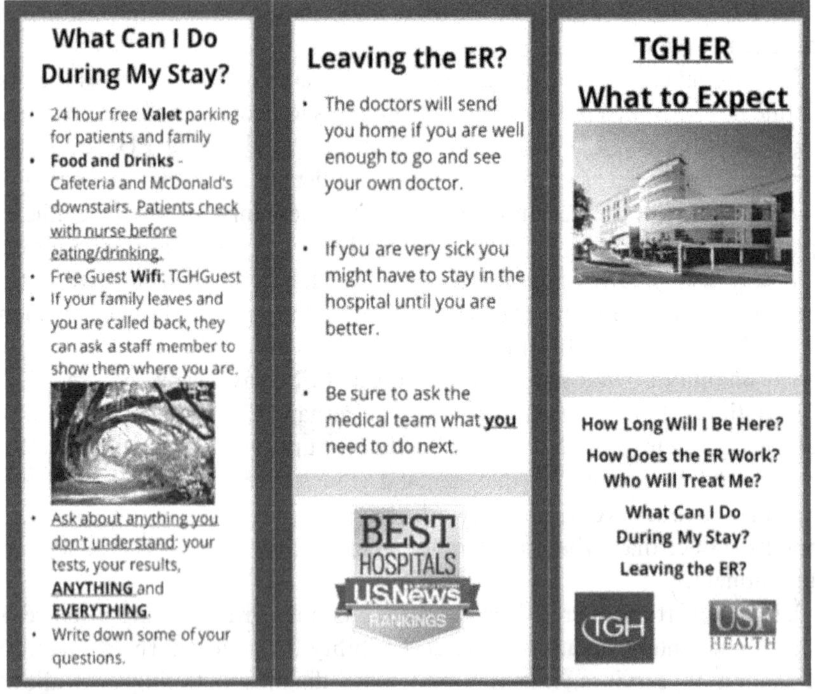

Figure 6.10 Front of the Leaflet that Was Created by the Class that Was Distributed to Patients in the ED at Registration.

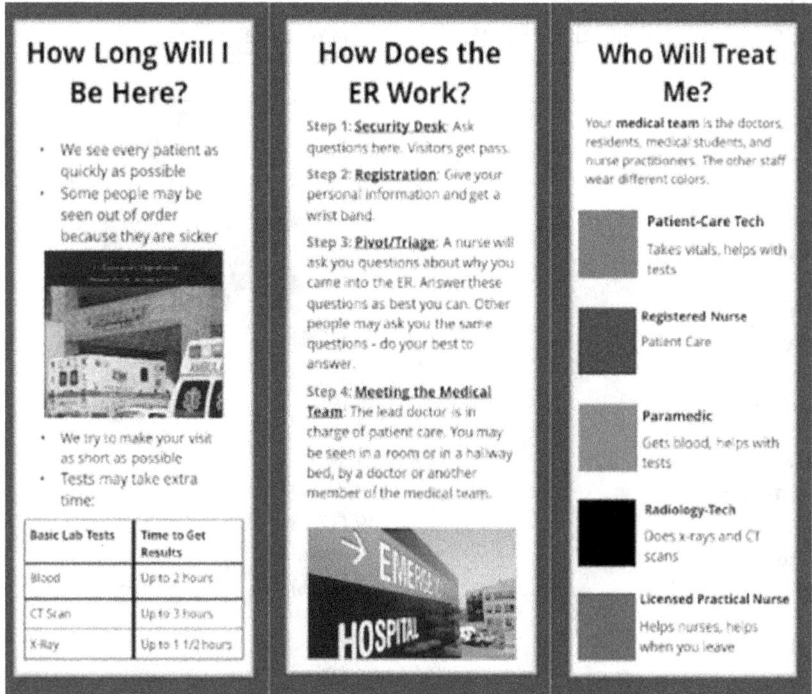

How Long Will I Be Here?

- We see every patient as quickly as possible
- Some people may be seen out of order because they are sicker
- We try to make your visit as short as possible
- Tests may take extra time:

Basic Lab Tests	Time to Get Results
Blood	Up to 2 hours
CT Scan	Up to 3 hours
X-Ray	Up to 1 1/2 hours

How Does the ER Work?

Step 1: **Security Desk**: Ask questions here. Visitors get pass.

Step 2: **Registration**: Give your personal information and get a wrist band.

Step 3: **Pivot/Triage**: A nurse will ask you questions about why you came into the ER. Answer these questions as best you can. Other people may ask you the same questions - do your best to answer.

Step 4: **Meeting the Medical Team**: The lead doctor is in charge of patient care. You may be seen in a room or in a hallway bed, by a doctor or another member of the medical team.

Who Will Treat Me?

Your **medical team** is the doctors, residents, medical students, and nurse practitioners. The other staff wear different colors.

Patient-Care Tech
Takes vitals, helps with tests

Registered Nurse
Patient Care

Paramedic
Gets blood, helps with tests

Radiology-Tech
Does x-rays and CT scans

Licensed Practical Nurse
Helps nurses, helps when you leave

Figure 6.11 Back of the Leaflet that Was Created by the Class that Was Distributed to Patients in the ED at Registration.

Analysis of data from over 200 interviews demonstrates that patients who received the class leaflet left the ED with fewer questions, a better understanding of their encounter, and a more complete picture of the ED. One 22-year-old white male patient described the leaflet as being "Nice, it's very good, thorough, well written, clean and simple, not too long to read." Another patient, a 60-year-old African American woman, stated, "I think it's very informational. Very helpful in my experience."

Positive patient responses were recorded in 64% of feedback interviews of patients who received the first version of the class designed leaflet. When our students asked patients, what was most helpful about the leaflet, 40% of respondents noted the description of the colors of the uniforms worn by different ED personnel (scrub colors equate to job roles and duties), 30% noted the clearer time expectations (diagnostic testing turnaround times), 15% noted creation of more clear general expectations, and 15% stated that it would only be helpful to patients who had not ever been in an ED on previous visits. The sentiment that the leaflet was more useful for those who had not been patients in the ED on previous encounters was heard in several interviews. One 59-year-old Hispanic female shared, "If today was my first time

Table 6.1 Demographics for Leaflet versus Non-leaflet Interviewees, Specifically Age, Sex, Education, and Whether They Were in a Room or a Hallway Bed.

	Non-Leaflet	*Leaflet*
Age		
18–39	41 (31%)	31 (40%)
40–59	51 (38%)	27 (35%)
>= 60	42 (31%)	20 (26%)
Mean Age	49.99	48.44
Gender		
Male	62 (46%)	34 (44%)
Female	66 (49%)	38 (46%)
Other/Missing	6 (4%)	6 (10%)
Education		
Less Than HS	18 (13%)	11 (14%)
HS/GED	49 (37%)	35 (32%)
Some College	30 (22%)	17 (22%)
BA/BS and Above	37 (28%)	25 (32%)
ED Location		
Hallway	28 (21%)	17 (22%)
Room	106 (79%)	61 (78%)
Sample Size	134	78

here it would have been [helpful]. I already know all this information, but I would have appreciated it during a previous visit."

Other critiques included the lack of clarification of how much time a patient should expect to spend in the waiting room before being taken back to a room. In addition, patients noted that while the leaflet was handed out at the front desk, no staff member encouraged the patient to review the leaflet. Patients who received the leaflet generally had a more positive feeling about ED staff, were clearer about how the ED works, had fewer low ratings of the ED. Overall, 90% of patients who received the initial leaflet stated that they liked the leaflet.

Interestingly, upon redesign of the leaflet by the hospital marketing team, there was a notable shift in the patient satisfaction with the new leaflet. There was a clear divide in patient satisfaction with both their care and with the leaflet overall immediately upon introduction of the new edition. These changes to the leaflet included a shift from fourth grade to college reading level, bright to muted colors, large blocks of text instead of smaller text blocks, and significantly fewer images. Images of the marketing form of the leaflet can be seen below in figures 6.12 and 6.13.

Table 6.2 Demographics for Leaflet versus Non-leaflet Interviewees, Specifically Ethnicity, First and Second Language (If Any).

	Non-Leaflet	*Leaflet*
Ethnicity/Self-Reported Race		
White	83 (62%)	41 (52%)
African American	17 (13%)	12 (15%)
Latinx/Hispanic	16 (12%)	10 (13%)
Asian	1 (0.1%)	3 (4%)
Missing	17 (12.9%)	3 (4%)
First Language		
English	115 (86%)	66 (86%)
Spanish	11 (9%)	10 (12%)
Other	5 (4%)	0 (0%)
Missing	3 (2%)	2 (2%)
Second Language		
English	16 (12%)	10 (13%)
Spanish	8 (6%)	5 (6%)
Other	6 (4%)	7 (9%)
None	101 (80%)	56 (71%)
Missing	3 (2%)	0 (0%)
Sample Size	134	78

These changes moved the leaflet further away from a patient-centric, patient data-driven product to a leaflet that more closely reproduced and served the branding and design needs of the marketing team, the organization, but not, necessarily, the patient. Patients who received the marketing version of the leaflet were notably less enthusiastic, in comparison to the patients who received the original version designed by the class.

When asked how the marketing leaflet could be improved, one 45-year-old Hispanic female patient stated, "Less wordy and even more pictures."

Comments of this type were seen in 40% of the interview responses about the marketing leaflet. The lack of pictures and the heavy emphasis on text was a common complaint about the second leaflet version that was initially approved by the marketing team. The increased reading level that the marketing team requested (demanded) was also a source of patient complaints. One patient, a 50-year-old white female stated, "More pictures, less words. My education [Bachelor's Degree] helped me read it."

This interviewee's response indicated that she believed that she was only able to read the leaflet because of her higher education and that reading the leaflet would be more challenging for people with less education. Compared

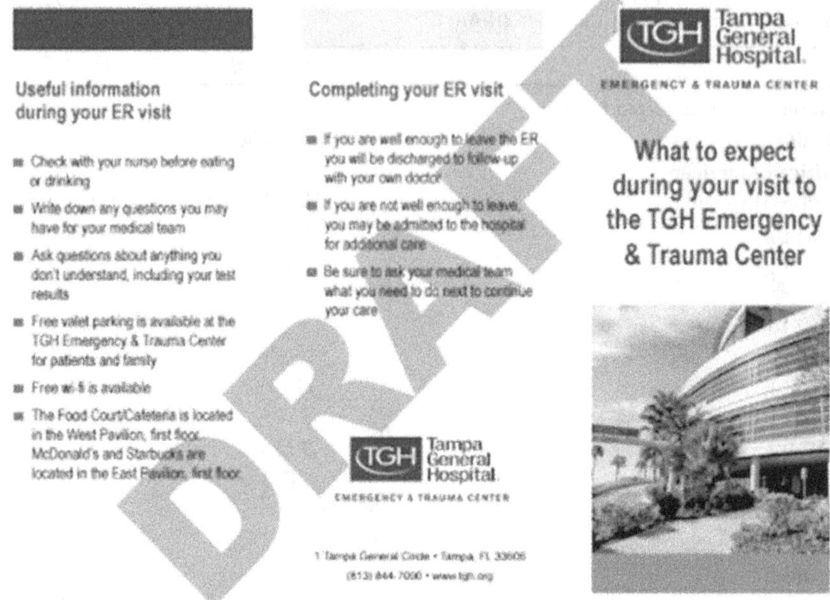

Figure 6.12 Front of the Leaflet that Was Created by the TGH Marketing Team that Was Distributed to Patients in the ED via Registration.

to no leaflet though, and despite the complaints, the marketing version of the leaflet was still successful, to an extent. Patients were generally more satisfied with their care and had clearer understandings of the ED upon discharge when they had the marketing version of the leaflet when compared to not having any form of material. However, patients who received the original form of the leaflet had the highest satisfaction and the best understanding of the ED of the three situations (no leaflet, class leaflet, marketing version of leaflet).

After the class project was presented, one-on-one stakeholder interviews continued, and collateral buy-in regarding the need to decrease the reading level of the leaflet was obtained from the hospital COO and patient experience director. All the individual stakeholder interviews have provided valuable insight into the thought processes of executives and other important people in the ED and across the hospital that are key to the permanent implementation of an ED leaflet. Even after leaflet distribution becomes hardwired, a continuous QI plan should be implemented to ensure that patient and stakeholder interviews continue to reshape the leaflet as new potential expectation mismatches arise.

Nevertheless, during this project, our students learned that it is imperative to find a way to both meet the expectations of these key stakeholders and

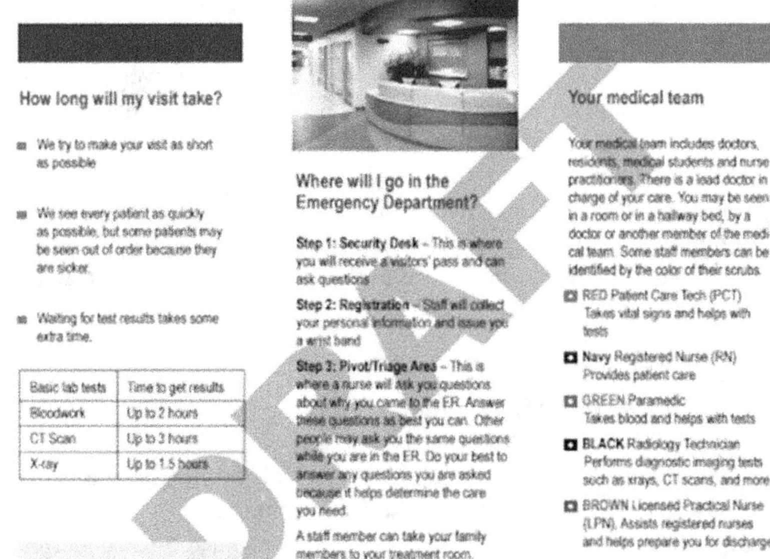

How long will my visit take?
We try to make your visit as short as possible
We see every patient as quickly as possible, but some patients may be seen out of order because they are sicker.
Waiting for test results takes some extra time.
Basic lab tests | Time to get results
Bloodwork | Up to 2 hours
CT Scan | Up to 3 hours
X-ray | Up to 1.5 hours
Where will I go in the Emergency Department?
Step 1: Security Desk – This is where you will receive a visitors' pass and can ask questions
Step 2: Registration – Staff will collect your personal information and issue you a wrist band
Step 3: Pivot/Triage Area – This is where a nurse will ask you questions about why you came to the ER. Answer these questions as best you can. Other people may ask you the same questions while you are in the ER. Do your best to answer any questions you are asked because it helps determine the care you need.
A staff member can take your family members to your treatment room.
Your medical team
Your medical team includes doctors, residents, medical students and nurse practitioners. There is a lead doctor in charge of your care. You may be seen in a room or in a hallway bed, by a doctor or another member of the medical team. Some staff members can be identified by the color of their scrubs.
RED Patient Care Tech (PCT) Takes vital signs and helps with tests
Navy Registered Nurse (RN) Provides patient care
GREEN Paramedic Takes blood and helps with tests
BLACK Radiology Technician Performs diagnostic imaging tests such as xrays, CT scans, and more
BROWN Licensed Practical Nurse (LPN). Assists registered nurses and helps prepare you for discharge
DRAFT

Figure 6.13 Back of the Leaflet that Was Created by the TGH Marketing Team that Was Distributed to Patients in the ED via Registration.

maintain the patient focus of the original leaflet. There is a natural tension that currently exists between these two views—whether that tension should exist is not entirely relevant at present. But it is interesting to imagine a healthcare system that more closely aligns a patient and organization centered approach to material creation. All the stakeholders did have their own role, responsibility, and desire to ensure hospital success, ED operational success, and certainly all hoped that patients would have a good experience. However, there were times when a good patient experience challenged other work product milestones and successes (e.g., a consistent and thematic branding pattern at a specific reading level showing organization savviness). All the interviewed stakeholders were supportive and interested in the project but struggled with implementation. Across the board, everyone understood the value of leaflets such as the one designed by the class, as well as the pros and cons of all the other examples that had been analyzed in the design phase of the class leaflet.

Ultimately, stakeholders and our thesis student (Kilian Kelly), along with both faculty (JWW and RDB), were able to reach an agreement that a successful leaflet should be presented at a lower reading level and that this would not damage brand reputation. In addition, we agreed on using low amounts of block text, bright colors, and copious images.

CONTRIBUTIONS TO THE ED

This project is not complete and, as of spring 2021, we were continuing to move through further refinements of final product, implementation, and standardized feedback stages. The shift in resources to hospital Covid-19 response during the spring of 2020 delayed the project as many ED processes changed during 2020–2021. We envision a future that merges patient and administrator concerns for the organization into an easier to negotiate shared perspective which will minimize care expectation mismatches and improve the patient experience.

THE ANTHROPOLOGICAL DIFFERENCE

This project demonstrates the value of medical anthropological data in addressing the mismatch between physician/hospital versus patient concepts of the role and functioning of the ED. The leaflet designed by an undergraduate class, based on anthropological qualitative research and data gathering (participant observation), was very successful in addressing patient concerns. However, this focus brought out several concerns from other stakeholders within the hospital. Nurses felt the description of them was too simplistic, while hospital marketing felt that the low reading level threatened the hospital image. What we have learned from this is that there are two approaches possible at this point. The first is to retreat from our patient-centered focus. The second path, which we are currently pursuing, is to educate those other stakeholders as to how they can leverage the use of a lower reading level to demonstrate the unique and progressive stance the hospital is taking to being patient centric, inclusive, and accessible to all. Our educational efforts, thus, must go beyond simply working with undergraduates (chapter 3), residents (chapter 5), and include all hospital stakeholders.

Chapter 7

Multi-Visit Patients

In the fall of 2018, Vizient (a large healthcare system benchmarking and performance improvement company, Vizient Inc. Dallas, Texas) initiated a multihospital project aimed at reducing Emergency Department (ED) visits and hospital encounters among patients who utilized hospital services the most. These patients (sometimes called frequent-fliers or, in more formal parlance, super-utilizers) are estimated to represent only a tiny fraction of the population but consume a highly disproportional share of healthcare resources while, paradoxically, not achieving improved healthcare outcomes. To establish corporate branding and identity for the Vizient project, that company used the term Multi-Visit Patients (MVPs) to describe the target population. The use of the acronym "MVP" also avoided any negative associations that patients may feel if labeled less positive associated terms such as frequent-flier.

The fall of 2018 was also the launch of our novel honors thesis class that RB and JW have taught once per year. The course consists of undergraduate students selected from the patient-physician interaction course (see chapter 3) and allows RB and JW to deliver didactic material to thesis students as a cohort, covering research design, ethics of research, and the development of an honors thesis research proposal for IRB submission at the end of the semester (with the student then spending the next semester conducting the proposed research). The novelty of the honors thesis course is that the projects are designed to allow our team to ask questions requiring a mixed methods approach and an applied medical anthropology lens to answer. For undergraduates, this is different than the common secondary data analysis often seen in many student theses. These projects place undergraduate pre-medical students directly into clinical settings, requiring the students to conduct participant observation as well as to spend time interviewing patients, physicians, and other healthcare workers. Ideally, students become engrained in the day-to-day rhythm of their clinical setting. This approach allows students to gain perspective from insiders and patients through these observations and interviews.

The Vizient MVP project was perfect for the involvement of an applied medical anthropologist and for a medical anthropology focused undergraduate honors thesis. Without the lens of anthropology, our hospital group, as part of the Vizient project, would generate data in terms of ICD-10 codes (billing codes used to classify disease at the end of a clinical encounter), throughput times (e.g., hospital length of stay), numbers of primary care visits in between hospital admissions, billing data, and patient outcome metrics but would be unlikely to elucidate patient-centered and patient-generated distributions of explanations for *why* they utilized our healthcare system so often. In addition, team members across the healthcare organization were able to contribute and assist in the Vizient project. The motivations, goals, and perspectives of team member participants could lead to improvement in similar projects by ensuring that program goals meshed with team members and vice versa in a way that leads to hardwired sustainability of any program wins (e.g., reduced utilization without decreasing healthcare outcome associated metrics).

There is a perception that the ED serves as a stand-in for patients to access primary care within the context of a broken healthcare system in the United States. If this perception is accurate, those with access to primary care will have fewer ED visits, have fewer hospital admissions, and utilize fewer healthcare resources. In reality, the difference between overall ED utilization between insured and uninsured patients is more complex. Some previous studies have suggested that patients with insurance may access healthcare service (including the ED) more often than uninsured patients (Zhou et al. 2017), although the implementation of the Affordable Care Act did lead to an overall decrease in ED visits by uninsured patients (Singer et al. 2019). If this sounds confusing, it is. The currently available quantitative data regarding healthcare utilization, spending, and outcomes are difficult to interpret.

BACKGROUND

The United States is also one of the few high-income countries without individual access to, or compulsory participation in, a single-payer healthcare system. Overall, the United States spends two to three times what other high-income countries spend as a percentage of GDP (around 18% in the United States compared to an average of 6.4% in other OECD countries, Health Statistics OECD). Federal, state, and local governments spend about $1.6 trillion on healthcare and, together, are the largest payer for healthcare

(NHE Fact Sheet, CMS). However, even though the U.S. government spends more on healthcare than other countries, all individuals in the United States do not have healthcare coverage and a number of healthcare outcomes used to measure the quality of health systems (e.g., mortality, life expectancy, birth weight) perform worse in the United States than in other countries. Interestingly, those with health insurance in the United States utilize more, not less, healthcare resources and those that visit the ED the most also visit their primary care providers more than other patients. People with Medicaid, a joint federal and state health insurance program, do utilize the ED more than other healthcare access points but do have access to primary care (Gathwaite et al. 2019). In other words, a review of quantitative data regarding healthcare outcomes and resource utilization in the United States presents several challenges to common assumptions and is difficult to interpret.

Mixed methods analysis holds value in adding texture and perspective to quantitative data that describes the "what" but not the "why." This methodological approach also presents a potential technique for moving past problems where more common approaches have left quantitative investigators stuck. Healthcare costs are still rising, and healthcare outcomes are still declining in the United States compared to other high-income countries, regardless of how much quantitative data we collect and analyze regarding spending, utilization, and outcomes in the United States. In other words, why does healthcare spending not track healthcare outcomes? Why do those with access to primary care visit the ED more often? Why do those that visit the ED more often also see their primary care doctor more than other similar patients controlled for health status, age, and other demographic variables?

One percent of the population spends approximately 25% of all healthcare dollars, while 5% of the population makes up 50% of healthcare spending in the United States (Healthsystemtracker.org, 2019). Is this from overutilization of resources? What is overutilization and what resources are we considering (diagnostic tests? ED visits? Hospital admissions? Home healthcare? Primary care visits?). When hearing that a small number of patients account for a disproportionate share of healthcare spending, we might assume that these are over-utilizers clogging up EDs with frivolous complaints or physicians over-testing those same over-utilizers secondary to fear of liability. Ethnographically, however, the story is different. At time of this writing, our ED, like many in the country, is at 70% capacity of beds utilized by patients admitted to the hospital for over four hours. Two-thirds of these patients have private health insurance. In other words, much of the crowding we see in EDs arrives secondary to a demand for the use of high revenue-generating hospital services behind the walls of the ED. Surgical procedures need postsurgical care and bed space, driving up demand and competition for beds that could be used by patients admitted from the ED. Instead, those ED patients often wait hours for a hospital bed owing partially to complex payment formula mixtures of inpatient and observation status revenue potential compared to surgical revenue. This does not mean those patients are less sick, but it does mean that there is a gamble, a probabilistic risk, of revenue for those patients compared to others (since one-third of ED patients may be underinsured or uninsured and some may be placed in observation status or have a long hospital length of stay—all factors that decrease revenue and create unpredictability compared to a surgical, procedural, or direct admission).

Reality is difficult to discern. Part of that spending is on acute disease states that require expensive treatment (e.g., cancer, trauma, infections leading to hospitalization, myocardial infarctions, and strokes). Breaking this down further, the members of the population in that 1% flow in and out, rarely staying at that high spending level for more than a year. This represents the underlying natural history of those high dollar disease states which either improve or lead to death. Population-level data are important to identify trends; however, qualitative patient-level interviews may provide context and insight into the data not available from quantitative analysis.

There is a paradigm shift in healthcare spending taking place in the United States. In the past, the system was designed to pay for quantity of care (fee-for-service) with little incentive to manage population health outcomes across groups of patients. As the federal government spends more on healthcare and takes on more risk, a push to increase the value of that spending has been implemented into current policy through "value-based purchasing" (CMS 2021). The concept of value-based purchasing is that healthcare spending should lead to improved outcomes. The concept of value has different meanings but, in current healthcare economics, can be represented as quality divided by cost (Value = Quality/Cost) where quality is the sum of healthcare outcomes and patient experiences.

The Centers for Medicare and Medicaid Services (CMS) is the largest payer of hospital services and hospital services make up a large percentage of overall healthcare spending. Thus, the federal government can operationalize value-based purchasing through CMS programs that lead to decreased Medicare reimbursements when spending does not track improvement in healthcare outcomes. Since Medicare spending represents a large percentage of hospital budgets, these institutions are vulnerable to decreases in Medicare reimbursements. To further incentivize participation in value-based care, institutions and physicians can also receive financial reward (increase reimbursement) when spending does lead to improved health outcomes through risk sharing arrangements known as Accountable Care Organizations (ACOs). To put this another way, hospital systems and provider groups that share risk must also manage population health, not just acute care episodes of patients in their networks as fee-for-service reimbursement decreases and becomes more restricted. Therefore, attention to nonmedical associated risk for hospital visits and poor health outcomes have received increased attention from entities and institutions that previously did not consider those so-called social determinants of health to be part of their scope.

Social determinants of health may include patient's income, housing status, substance use, mental health, domestic violence victim status or ongoing abuse, migrant or refugee documentation status, employment/employment history, gender, sexual orientation, access to reliable transportation, caregiver responsibilities, and other structural forces that mitigate when and where a patient seeks care as well as the ability for a patient to follow a care plan, change behaviors, or take medications that directly influence healthcare outcomes. Medicine and public health commonly use the term "social determinants," broadly lumping these structural problems under a category of health determination that is not seen to fall neatly within a box of genetic risk or medical history. Social scientists might be more familiar with the term "structural" determinants and that term does allow better categorization of these risk factors and places less individual blame while also assigning less agency to these risk factors as being relegated to a tangential space outside of medicine and the responsibility of the patient to fix by better navigating their social space. These structural forces that explain where and when a patient seeks care, as well as healthcare outcomes (probably even more so than medical risk factors), are part of an everyday assault on a patient's overall wellbeing and health that has been called structural violence (Farmer et al. 2006).

Previously, medicine looked to public health and social science to consider population health. However, the shift to value-based purchasing has relegated responsibility for population health management back to providers and hospitals that might have previously focused instead on individual physician-patient encounters or acute episodes of disease. The shift to value-based purchasing and the requirement to manage population health even at the provider and institution level necessitates a focus on everyday structural violence in the lives of patients that previously lacked significant focus in healthcare.

The perception that EDs are filled with patients seeking primary care for frivolous complaints is overblown and does not mirror reality. EDs in the United States care for approximately 70% of unscheduled and acute encounters but spending in the ED represents only 2% of all healthcare dollars (ACEP). In 2017, there were 145.6 million ED encounters, representing 45.8 visits per 100 persons (CDC). However, the focus on ED utilization remains important when considering ways to decrease cost and ED visits also serve as a barometer on population health management. ED encounters lead to admission about 10% of the time. Hospital admission is the most expensive decision a physician can make and costs the healthcare system over $11,700 (or about $381 billion per year) (HCUP 2020). An ACO or physician group participating in a risk sharing model requires a population health approach. When a patient ends up in the ED with a 10% chance of admission, the risk of a positive net margin begins to dissipate rapidly, especially if a patient has multiple ED encounters in each billing period.

In other words, the 10% chance of hospital admission from the ED is not an independent event but instead increases each time the patient visits the ED as the return visit may signal that an outpatient treatment plan failed or a pathway for follow-up was not available and the patient is becoming sicker, increasing health risk to that patient, and potentially in the United States, increasing medicolegal risk to the treating provider. Therefore, ED utilization and hospital admissions have been the primary focus of most super-utilizer programs aimed at reducing per patient spending and healthcare cost to date.

The 1979 satire novel *The House of God* (written by psychiatrist Stephen Bergman under the pen name Samuel Shem) cemented the term "GOMER" (Get Out of My ER) to describe patients that visited the ED and hospital so frequently that hospital staff knew the patients' names and personal history as though it was a primary care office (Shem 1979). These GOMERs are often presented in *The House of God* (and in reality) with complex, intertwined life and medical problems that might include a chronic medical condition, such as coronary artery disease, within the context of homelessness, recent incarceration, poverty, and, often, mental illness as well.

While the term "GOMER" was (and sometimes, quietly, still is) used by frontline healthcare staff, the recognition that the term could be perceived with negative connotations led to the development of friendlier sounding phrases such as "frequent-flier" which is currently the most common informal way that frontline healthcare workers (i.e., nurses, paramedics, and doctors but not administration) still refer to those individuals that visit well above the average number of times of another patient. Frequent-flier certainly is less loaded than GOMER but does not have the proper parlance needed within the neoliberal framework of healthcare consumers and suppliers. More recently, the term "super-utilizer" has gained ground in the medical literature capturing both the process and problem encapsulated in these types of patients from the viewpoint of the healthcare system and overall healthcare spending.

Precise definitions of super-utilizer are not clear but usually are based on a threshold number of visits per year to an ED, or several admissions per year to a hospital. For example, one system may define a super-utilizer as any patient that visits the ED more than four times per year or has more than two hospital admissions per year. In an academic, tertiary care center though, this might be the median for the patient population or simply represent patients that have chronic disease that, even when managed well, will intermittently result in exacerbations and acute emergencies. Other systems create multiple tiers for patients. Super-utilizers may represent a standard deviation above the mean patient encounter number but "high super-utilizers" may represent 2 or 3 times the standard deviation, maybe more than 12 ED encounters per year. The definition is important for a healthcare system to agree on as this is often how resources are targeted for intensive case management and other strategies aimed at decreasing utilization. The term "super-utilizer" also hints at the solution—namely, to decrease utilization of healthcare resources among these patients. Since ED encounters can lead to hospital admissions and hospital admissions are the highest cost resource, it is reasonable that approaches to decrease super-utilizer costs often focus on decreasing ED visits.

Mark Fleming, an anthropologist at the University of California, San Francisco, (UCSF), along with a team of other social scientists and public health workers, considered the neoliberal context of increased emphasis on super-utilizers access to the healthcare system (Fleming et al. 2017). In Fleming's research, his team conducted ethnographic fieldwork among an interdisciplinary hospital group aimed at reducing utilization by super-utilizers throughout the UCSF hospital and primary care system. Not surprisingly, the target population had multiple medical and social comorbidities that were difficult to unravel from each other including homelessness, mental health, and chronic medical disease problems that appeared to be in poor control even after paradoxical high utilization of healthcare. This paradox of high utilization but worse healthcare outcomes is common among super-utilizer populations both in Fleming's work and in other studies examining these groups of patients (UPMC). Derek, a community healthcare worker interviewed by Fleming, described this paradox as "over serviced but under-served" (Fleming et al. 2017).

Fleming found that the interdisciplinary care team focused on a need to demonstrate to hospital administration that their efforts would result in a positive return on investment (ROI). We have found, like these researchers, that hospital administrators have difficulty envisioning perceived cost savings from reduced visits but instead want to see actual revenue generation or measurable cost reductions. The lack of revenue generation means that positive ROI would show up in measurable cost reduction in value-based purchasing-related metrics or savings in state or federal payments to the hospital to cover low-income patients. The emphasis on low-income patients in consideration of superutilizer populations is worth unpacking.

Most super-utilizer projects, including the UCSF project, exclude those patients that have multiple visits secondary to terminal conditions, cancer, or subacute care episodes that may be known to take one to two years to resolve either in resolution or in death. It turns out that excluding those patient groups often leaves a group of low-income, underinsured patients. Through this selective bias, what the teams focusing on reducing super-utilizer encounters are often left with are some of the most challenging patients to demonstrate positive ROI: end-stage renal disease on hemodialysis (often undocumented without the ability to obtain federal funding to pay for dialysis services), patients with concomitant diabetes and coronary artery disease, patients with hepatitis C virus infection, substance abuse, chronic pain, and multiple mental health diagnoses including schizophrenia and bipolar. Underinsured status and poverty are often common variables across these groups of patients. Interestingly, in a few studies (UPMC [Bryk et al. 2018], CARES [Bronsky et al. 2018], Fleming et al. [2017]), there are often more white women represented than any other group of people (about 60% across multiple studies).

This difficulty in demonstrating ROI has, in the past, led to neglect of care plans for these patients that did not generate at least potential or small revenue in the fee-for-service model. Medicaid may not reimburse much but it does reimburse something, often leading to repeated procedures for repeated complaints (e.g., colonoscopy for the chronic abdominal pain patient who has crowded housing, poor diet, and substance use).

Perhaps, as suggested back in the late 1970s, much of these repeated visits can be attributed to a mismatch in seeking care for illness by the patient versus trying to provide care for disease by physicians and healthcare teams (Kleinman et al. 1978). Perhaps all of our interventions to decrease high-cost utilization simply reproduce the same structured models and maintain the same clinical distances, resulting in no change in care or utilization outcomes.

The Camden, New Jersey "hot spotter" approach is an intensive, data-driven, method of identifying super-utilizer patients and intervening to help guide those patients to perceived less costly care environments—that is, a clinic instead of the ED, a tele visit instead of a clinic—using face-to-face care navigators (Finkelstein et al. 2020). The hot spotter program received wide attention when best-selling author and New Yorker writer and physician Atul Gawande covered the project in one of his columns (Gawande 2011). Certainly, if intensive case management/navigator interventions could lead to decreases in high-cost utilization for a disproportionately small number of patients, this was going to be the program that would show an ROI. Unfortunately, data published in the *New England Journal of Medicine* in 2020 did not show positive results of the best designed, largest specific trial to reduce cost in care for super-utilizers.

Jeffrey Brenner, also featured in the article by Gawande, was the principal investigator of the hot spotting trial that was initially designed in 2014. Camden is an economically depressed area (37% below poverty line) with a sick and vulnerable patient population. As mentioned previously, one of the difficulties in distinguishing positive or negative trial results or summarizing super-utilizer studies is that many of the projects still use different definitions of super-utilizer. There is some appropriateness to this given that different healthcare systems may have different distributions of utilization, with high utilization meaning something different at two different places. As an aside, a federally supported (e.g., CMS, AHCA, or CDC) definition and defined throughput metric for this concept would be helpful in both benchmarking across healthcare systems and designing research studies. Groups like Vizient have worked to standardize metrics by first understanding the patient population treated at a given healthcare facility, recognizing some systems may care for sicker patients than others. Using those data, Vizient has been able to mathematically adjust comparisons to formulate observed to expected metric concepts based on specific disease states or types of hospitals (e.g., comparing teaching hospitals to each other). Groups like Vizient could turn attention to super-utilizers to establish better across system comparison standards.

In the Camden study, super-utilizers were defined as any patient with at least one hospital admission in the prior six months plus concomitant presence of at least two chronic conditions and simultaneous presence of another two high-risk traits including five active medications, difficulty accessing services, lack of social support, a coexisting mental health condition, active illicit drug use, or homelessness (Brenner et al. 2014). Patients enrolled in the hot-spotting Camden trial had some type of insurance of government-supported payment (e.g., Medicaid) and were not being treated for active cancer (a common exclusion criteria with its own set of problems for why we exclude this disease state but not others such as substance use that might also have a finite treatment course if treated as disease). In the Camden study, study participants accounted for less than 0.5% of the hospital system population but utilized 11% of the resources.

The hot spotter program utilized home care managers to assist the experimental arm participants with face-to-face visits. During these visits, care managers helped patients complete healthcare navigation tasks, enroll in social service programs and healthcare benefit plans, make follow-up appointments, get to those appointments, and complete preventive care tasks (such as checking blood glucose and blood pressure). The hot spotter concept refers to the targeting of intense interventions to areas within the Camden system that are, essentially in real time, witnessing high service use (i.e., large readmission rates).

The control arm in the Camden study received standard of care, which often consists of printed discharge instructions after a hospital encounter. There were 800 participants in the study (399 in the treatment group and 401 in the control group). The primary outcome that the study was powered to detect was a 9% decrease in admission rates at 180 days in the treatment arm (Brenner et al. 2014).

During the study, patients in the treatment arm underwent over 7 home visits and over 8 phone calls from study case manager staff during a median participation time of 92 days. Rates of federal assistance acquisition (SNAP and TANF) were low in both arms and not statistically significantly higher in the treatment arm at the end of the trial. In addition, the readmission rate was about 62% in both arms—no statistical difference. While some prior intervention programs targeted at Medicare patients have seen decreases of 15% to 45% in the readmission rate, this study had a younger (mean age range 45 to 64 years old) sample with potentially more comorbidities and social determinants of health. While decreasing utilization of services in Medicare patients might lead to decreased ROI, the significant disproportional representation of 0.5% of Camden patients accounting for 11% of spending should not be dismissed. In other words, to make a scalable impact on ROI with decreased healthcare spending, showing treatment affects in younger populations will be needed—which may mean that the social determinants of care have an even higher impact on overall care management and health outcome metrics than originally expected. Perhaps if the treatment arm would have had increased rates of SNAP and TANF that would have led to differences in healthcare outcomes? The NEJM study is critically important because this trial was nationally seen as the "right" way to go about addressing super-utilizers, was well funded, had a case control experimental design, had input of multiple experts, and had received publicity. Unfortunately, the medical model for decreasing utilization failed. Furthermore, while the NEJM article shows us quantitatively that this was a negative study—that is, no statistically significant difference in readmission rates between the two arms—we do not have any specific patient (or provider/staff) level insight into why.

The goal of our project was to utilize a mixed methods approach to complement quantitative data collected during a hospital benchmarking period of a subset of super-utilizers as well as to capture patient-level feedback on why they chose to access healthcare when, where, and how they were observed doing (often with frequent visits to the ED leading to hospital admissions). Our study design allows for gathering of patient generated feedback into why specific super-utilizer interventions might fail, succeed or be abandoned for a different focus or approach altogether.

METHODS

Our hospital participated in a multi-institution Vizient initiative to decrease high costs associated with super-utilizer patients, called multi-visit patients, or MVPs in the project. First, key stakeholders met for a webinar led by Vizient to understand project goals. Next, that group again met to outline our target population as well as to identify other key stakeholders who might be needed for project success but were not yet present at the meetings. After identification of our MVP target population, we worked with our hospital IT department to ensure that any time an MVP entered the hospital, our team would be notified. Our hospital uses a system-wide electronic medical record (Epic) in which our IT department was able to create a daily automated list of the MVP patients. Next, we decided on what our first phase goal would be and decided to conduct a multidisciplinary patient needs and perspective analysis. More specifically, our goal was to engage each targeted MVP patient and conduct an interview with a social work student or social worker using a semi-structured interview guide. In addition, an honors thesis student that had taken the Research in Patient-Physician Interaction course and was enrolled in the honors thesis course (see chapter 3) would also interview as many targeted MVP patients as possible, adding to the data collected by the social worker. Each day, a larger team of physicians, social workers, as well as process improvement and Quality Improvement (QI) specialists would review interview data and then meet weekly to formulate care plans for the patient based on patient-generated needs from the interview data. JWW served as both a committee member physician for the hospital MVP QI project and the thesis adviser, along with RDB, for Meera Navadia, the undergraduate student that conducted some of the interviews reported here for her honors thesis. The analysis of the data presented here is from participant observation field notes of JWW and MN as well as social work interview notes and interview notes from interviews conducted by MN. After data collection, graduate student Emily Holbrook coded the data, identifying thematic codes. MN independently coded data from her interview participants and then compared those themes to the themes identified from the other interview data coded by EH to increase the sample size and to identify larger themes that emerged during coding. Unfortunately, the MVP project coordinated by Vizient was only a six-month pilot and most institutions did not move into data analysis phase during this time. Thus, our hospital suspended staff support of the project after the completion of the Vizient time frame. However, the automated MVP list continued to be generated and MN continued to conduct target MVP interviews throughout the fall of 2019. This project was a hospital-wide QI project, and there was no specific intervention arm. Thus, there were no human subjects and IRB review was not required.

Our hospital has multiple hospitalist groups (internal medicine physicians that admit patients to the hospital), but the largest group accounting for most hospital admissions is the University of South Florida (USF) Internal Medicine service. Thus, we chose the USF Internal Medicine team as the MVP target group. We then examined the distribution of patient admissions and focused on the 90th percentile of admissions to further refine our target population (here, patients with > = 4 admissions to the hospital in the baseline period. Next, we excluded patients with a cancer-related diagnosis. Interestingly, cancer-related diagnoses are often excluded from this type of study, but should they be included? Is there a reason we create an environment of expectation of high utilization for the cancer patient but not for other patient disease states associated with subacute time frames of high resource use? Either way, we next excluded patients with Medicare as this represents a different population and potentially other strategies for resource utilization refinement. In other words, Medicare patients are older and often have diagnosed chronic disease states or known end of life issues. Interventions focused on those chronic disease states may be more medical than the intended project goals (i.e., congestive heart failure compared to mental illness). Patients admitted to the hospital in law enforcement custody or under a current psychiatric legal hold were also excluded (although patients with chronic mental illness were included). After we arrived at a target population, we provided these parameters to our IT team and an automated report was built and began to be distributed by email each morning. The average number of patients on the list on any given day (mean) was 8 and the number of new patients (i.e., patients that were not on the list the previous day) was 2 while the length of stay for these patients was longer than the hospital average (5.9 days compared to 5.5 days).

Each morning, an MVP Report was sent out to the team, including the student Meera Nevadia. Working with JWW, the social workers and case managers, and the hospitalists, patients were chosen for further interviews either secondary to convenience or lack of clarity around why the patient had presented to the hospital multiple times after review of the medical record. Social work students and case managers, as well as Meera, all conducted interviews.

Social work student interviews often first focused on the medical history, then the number of admissions in the past year, then ways that the patient accessed care outside of the hospital or managed their disease at home. Working with RDB and JWW, Meera instead focused on more open-ended approaches to the interview questions with MVP patients.

Following verbal consent, open-ended questions were utilized with a mix of semi-structured questions. A free list approach was used for participants to consider their view of what constitutes a good care experience at Tampa General. Participants that had a behavioral health diagnosis were also prompted to about how that diagnosis affected their healthcare access.

We reviewed 13 interviews conducted by Meera Nevadia as part of this project and analyzed those interviews for themes. The semi-structured interview is located below.

PATIENT INTERVIEW

1. Why did you come to the hospital today?
2. What health problems do you have? What health problems have your doctors talked to you about?

   a. If no behavioral illnesses are mentioned, questions will proceed to Question 4.
   b. If behavioral illnesses are mentioned questions will be followed up with additional questions below before moving forward to Question 4.
      i. Did you know anything else about your illness?
      ii. How did your family react to the news?
      iii. What was the first thing that came to your mind, when you were told about your condition?
3. Tell me how you felt when you were told about your health problem?
4. Have symptoms gotten worse or better with time?
5. Do you have a primary care physician?
6. Do you have any issues with transportation to the hospital or other medical facilities?
7. Tell me about any problems you must get medical help.
8. What do you believe is the hardest part of taking care of yourself and health?
9. Why do you choose to visit the ED, compared to going to the doctor's office?
10. What can Tampa General Hospital and staff help you with?

The semi-structured interview conducted by our team is different than the SW/CM model that utilized a template for medical history, number of visits, primary care access, funding status, and a psychosocial assessment including patient perceived barriers to care including mental illness, transportation, and domestic family issues. Chart review was used to corroborate patient-reported medical data and responses.

RESULTS

Overall, the number of interviews conducted and the level of experience of the interviewer (e.g., lack of probing questions) did not allow for a clear saturation point among the sample when the interviews were thematically analyzed. The 13 interviews consisted of 8 male and 5 female participants. Ten of those participants were white and three were African American. All spoke English as their primary language. The youngest person interviewed was 27 years old and the oldest person was 98 (a potentially problematic age range when considering common themes for multiple visits). The hospital length of stay in this cohort ranged from 4 to 20 days.

Interestingly, access to a primary physician was not a theme that arose for most of the patients and 61% of the patients reported having an established primary care physician that they could see when needed. While the thematic analysis of this data lacked other clear themes, there were some important insights gained from the qualitative data. For example, one elderly patient reported that they come to the hospital so often because they like the company, while another patient had insight into the existence of both illness and disease as reasons for care seeking. Exemplary patient quotes are found in table 7.1.

Eighty percent of patients reported that they access care at the ED not because they could not obtain care outside of the hospital but, instead, because care in the ED was quick, convenient, and easier to access. Sixty-one percent of the patients interviewed also had a reported substance use disorder or history of mental illness, including major depressive disorder. Unfortunately, likely secondary to the experience of the student interviewer, these patients were not willing to discuss those disorders in much detail. The student felt that the most important trends were not lack of primary care access, lack of transportation, or lack of health insurance (only 1 patient reported transportation issues, 61% had a primary care physician, and, per chart review, and 76% of participants had at least Medicaid level funding). Medicaid, a federal state–funded source for healthcare payments, does provide reimbursement for hospital and primary care visits. However, the number of specialists that accept Medicaid is limited. Thus, specialty care may require multi-month waits and limited encounters each year. All 13 patients reported at least 1 chronic medical condition (diabetes, pancreatitis, congestive heart failure). While lack of insurance may not have been the driving factor for repeated hospital visits, long-term high-quality chronic care management with specialist physicians might be limited outside of the acute care setting secondary to the underinsured status often associated with Medicaid and other indigent care local health funding programs (e.g., Hillsborough County Healthcare Plan).

Table 7.1 MVP Quotes Regarding Their Own Perceptions of Multiple Hospital Encounters.

"Sickle cell is not a joke, people do not understand, you cannot have a job, you cannot have a normal life due to this illness"
—37-year-old African American male patient with sickle cell anemia
"Physicians should treat the patient not the monitor"
—43-year-old, white, female patient receiving DHE treatment
"Cure my illness, and that will reduce my visits"
—59-year-old, African American, male patient with pancreatitis
"It is a terrible feeling lonely, I come to the hospital to enjoy some company"
—90-year-old, white, female patient for chronic kidney and heart disease
"It is just something you have to go through in life"
—50-year-old, white, male patient on list for heart transplant

The most interesting insights came from interdisciplinary team interviews and engagement with one specific patient, referred to here by pseudonym Susan Smith.

SUSAN SMITH

Susan Smith has a known history of insulin-dependent diabetes, pancreatitis (an intermittent, reoccurring inflammation of the pancreas), and borderline personality disorder. A 46-year-old white woman from Florida, she was included in the MVP project secondary to her 38 hospital admissions over a 12-month period.

The patient presented 72 times to the ED in one year. Many times, the complaints focused on generalized body pain or abdominal pain and were felt to be part of a complicated regional pain syndrome, inherent to her borderline personality disorder, and/or potentially psychosomatic. The patient had previously seen a chronic pain management specialist but, per the patient, did not feel that this was needed any longer. She had no definitive history of opioid abuse, had never been admitted or had an encounter for an opioid overdose, and prior urine drug screens did not identify any other substances. At times, the patient's pain was associated with elevated glucose levels.

The glucose levels were markedly elevated, and the patient had ketones in her blood. Ketones are evidence for a metabolic process described as ketonuria and indicative that the body was not getting enough insulin to utilize consumed sugars. These ketones are an acid and high levels of ketones can lead to a potentially deadly acute disease state called diabetic ketoacidosis (DKA). At times, Ms. Smith was in DKA. Other times, she simply had high glucose levels but no ketones (hyperglycemia). The encounters often led to admission given the high risk of progression to DKA with her hyperglycemia and the high risk of poor outcomes when in acute DKA.

Social workers attempted to ensure that Ms. Smith had appropriate transport to and from her outpatient physician office, that she had appropriate funding to pay for her insulin, and that she was getting her medications prescribed and knew where to pick them up.

Ms. Smith was known to have a primary care physician in a nearby town, approximately 40 miles from Tampa (Brooksville, Florida). Discussions with that physician verified that she did attend some of her primary care appointments with a follow-up rate of about 50% of the time. That physician prescribed the patient's insulin. Phone calls to a retail pharmacy in Brooksville confirmed that the patient had regularly filled the prescription. Why was Ms. Smith coming all the way to Tampa, bypassing at least 5 other hospitals in the 40-mile drive south down I-75?

If Ms. Smith had a primary care doctor, why did she utilize a hospital that was 40 miles away so often?

Ms. Smith had been interviewed multiple times by our case management team. However, JWW conducted several patient interviews to help facilitate the work of the honors thesis student. We asked Ms. Smith why she traveled so far for her care and her explanation was revealing:

Ms. Smith: Other hospitals won't do anything. No one talks to me about any of this stuff. Sometimes they admit me, sometimes they send me home. But they never do anything for me. This hospital always does something for me, even when everyone is mad at me.

JWW: Why do you think everyone is mad at you?

Ms. Smith: Because I don't take any of my medicines, I get sick, and I end up back here.

JWW: You don't take your medicines? Your insulin?

Ms. Smith: Nope. Hardly ever.

JWW: Can you not afford it? Can you not get it?

Ms. Smith: I have it. They give me more every time I come. I have pens and pens, boxes of the stuff.

JWW: What did you mention to the social worker about your religion last time? [The patient had been placed on a psychiatric hold previously and stated she was Catholic and that it was silly of us to think that she would attempt suicide.]

Ms. Smith: Yeah, I told that I'm a devout Catholic. I mean, come on, my whole family came from Ireland. I was the first person born here. They are really serious and my dad is still alive. I really want to die but I can't kill myself. Eventually though, diabetes will kill me.

JWW: Is that why you don't take you medications? So that diabetes can kill you?

Ms. Smith: I can't kill myself.

DISCUSSION AND CONTRIBUTIONS OF ANTHROPOLOGY

The potentiality of a mixed methods approach to better understanding super-utilizers suggests that medical anthropologists might be able to play their most important role around healthcare issues in which traditional approaches have led to stagnate outcomes or marginal improvements. Patient-informed data allows for myth-shattering revelations (e.g., perhaps frequent ED encounters are not secondary to lack of primary care in this population, or, perhaps, a patient is not compliant with medications not secondary to financial or education issues but instead underlying psychiatric depression) as well as hidden motivations not seen by quantitative data analysis or other forms of interview (e.g., the traditional social work biopsychosocial assessment). As we continue to refine the coordinated curriculum and deployment of medical anthropologists across the healthcare space, we will consider the lessons learned from the MVP project. This was a challenging project for a nascent premedical student without a primary focus in social science. While we certainly believe that a premedical student, especially after our undergraduate course, could participate and engage in a complex mixed methods project, we also think that this type of project would work better as part of a team that includes graduate-level anthropology students, medical students with patient experience, and possibly resident physicians all led by an experienced physician or anthropologist.

Further examples of utilizing anthropological approaches to "get at" stagnate healthcare problems in a different way are covered in chapters 8, 10, and 11 when we discuss work on opioid use disorder (10), patients with sickle cell disease (8), and patients that present to the ED after gunshot wound injury (11). Those projects have involved more experienced researchers alongside premedical undergraduates and longitudinal in nature, allowing time for refinement in the methodological approach.

Chapter 8

Sickle Cell Disease

Contributions by Carlos Osorno-Cruz

Our work in the Emergency Department (ED) with Sickle Cell Disease (SCD) patients provides an example of how mixed methods can lead to applied anthropological contributions relevant to clinical partners by demonstrating ways that patient care can be improved through the integration of patient-specific concerns and best treatment practices. Like our work with opioid use disorder and HCV, new ways of managing patients with SCD-related pain in the ED provides another example of how we use medical anthropology to construct new patient care pathways while also participating in the education of healthcare providers.

The most common reason for patients with SCD to present to the ED is secondary to pain. Previously, SCD patients who presented to the Tampa General Hospital (TGH) ED were often unsatisfied with their experiences, remained in pain throughout the duration of their encounter and were frequently admitted to the hospital secondary to unmet expectations of the patient, leading to patient and provider frustration. Provider frustration arose from lack of available tools to meet patient expectations, distrust of the patient's motives and reasons for coming to the ED (pain from disease or pain from malingering), and previous experiences with SCD patients in which the encounter often did not go well and the patient demonstrated little improvement over the course of multiple hours in the department. In other words, hospital admission, while sometimes necessary in SCD patients, resulted in the ED out of frustration that the patient was still in pain, unhappy, and with the ED provider feeling that nothing more could be done to improve the situation.

BACKGROUND

The SCD initiative discussed here was a mixed methods quality improvement project that also involved a premedical anthropology student (Carlos Osorno) working alongside a medical resident (Alex Nappi, MD) and an attending physician (JWW) in a clinical space—illustrating how both anthropologists might be deployed into this type of space and also how patient-centered projects for premedical students can shift the clinical gaze over the long term as Carlo Osorno is, as of this writing, a third-year medical student at the University of Iowa.

Patients with SCD who present to the ED in vaso-occlusive crises (VOC) have unmet expectations secondary to inconsistent implementation of evidence-based approaches to pain management, the subjective nature of pain, and stigma associated with opioid dependence. Historical patterns of slavery, Jim Crow Laws, and other forms of structural racism in the U.S. south also complicate relationships between mostly white caregivers and mostly black patients. Without clear pathways and shared physician-patient expectations, there is significant chance that mismatched expectations and stigma will lead to poor patient experience.

SCD

African Americans represent the majority of the 100,000 patients with SCD in the United States secondary to the slave trade that brought many people with the hemoglobin-S (Hb-S) gene variant to the country over 200 years ago. One out of 365 black or African American births has SCD compared to 1 out of every 16,300 Hispanic-American births. There is a higher prevalence of SCD in equatorial areas, including south Asia and Sub-Saharan Africa secondary to a relationship between the prevalence of SCD and the incidence of malaria resulting from *Anopheles* mosquito transmission of Plasmodium.

SCD results from a genetic disorder (Hb-SS) that affects hemoglobin (the protein that carries oxygen in red blood cells) and results in abnormally shaped red blood cells. Without access to medical care, humans with SCD live much shorter lives than those without disease or those with the heterozygote trait. Thus, the fitness (realization of reproductive potential) in patients with Hb-SS (the homozygote recessive genetic signature of SCD) is greatly reduced. Incidentally, the shape of sickled cells also inhibits the life cycle of Plasmodium and creates an inhibitory environment for the parasite. Thus, people with SCD or Sickle Cell Trait have lower incidence of malaria. Given that those with Sickle Cell Trait are protected from mortality associated with malaria, the Hb-S gene has retained prevalence in those populations in equatorial regions with a high incidence of malaria.

Patients with SCD will eventually experience emergent conditions during acute crises in which large volumes of sickled cells clump together, blocking vasculature and leading to end organ damage or infarct. SCD patients may present to the ED while undergoing an emergent medical condition (EMC). Emergent conditions in patients with SCD include acute chest syndrome, pneumonia, osteomyelitis (bone infection), bacteremia (blood stream infection), or even stroke. In addition, SCD patients undergo inevitable splenic infarct (placing them at higher risk for infection from encapsulated organisms) as well as avascular necrosis (death and loss of bone from decreased delivery of oxygenated blood).

Patients with SCD begin interaction with biomedicine in the United States at a very young age. These interactions with Western Medicine are often secondary to pain and suffering but also in the context of the downstream emergent sequelae of VOC. Unfortunately, even when not experiencing an EMC, patients with SCD suffer from daily micro-occlusion events within the venous system that may be less threatening to end organs but cause pain from disruption of normal blood return. If these events are worse than usual, they may be considered VOC and require aggressive medical management of the resulting pain. The daily nature of SCD pain, coupled with intermittent peaks of VOC, results in a dependence on medication (often powerful opioids) to manage symptoms. Therefore, patients with SCD suffer from chronic pain syndromes and are at constant risk for medical emergencies. Many patients with SCD can control their pain utilizing oral medications; however, when acute on chronic exacerbations of pain occur, many SCD patients seek care in the ED for relief of suffering. Emergency Medicine (EM) physicians are trained to rule out EMCs by completing a medical screening exam (MSE) and receive little training in the management of chronic pain syndromes. The approach to ruling out an EMC across physicians is similar but, after an EMC is ruled out, a high degree of variability exists in approaches to pain management.

SCD VOD, PAIN, AND BIAS

An acute chronic pain syndrome may be from true VOC but also may be part of a more complicated opioid dependence disorder. There are no objective criteria for VOC that has been validated, and the degree of current pain is a subjective reflection of suffering. In the United States, patients with SCD that survive to adulthood are often managed with opioid medications, often at doses like patients with terminal cancer. At some point, physiological dependence on opioids develops. Stigma surrounding chronic pain syndromes and opioid dependence may mitigate aggressive pain management in the ED in the context of focus on EMCs, stigma, deservingness, structural racism, implicit bias, and lack of training in the management of these conditions. The subjective nature of SCD-related pain creates context in which an EM physician must believe the verbal expression of pain expressed by a suffering SCD patient. Many ED physicians treating patients with VOC feel unprepared, undertrained, and, overall, not responsible for the management of chronic conditions, increasing the variability in approaches to patients with SCD-related pain. This variability leads to unmet patient expectations.

SCD, PATIENT EXPERIENCE, PATIENT SATISFACTION

Most of the EDs in the United States that care for a large volume of SCD patients are in the southeast, mirroring post-reconstruction settlement areas of African Americans in the United States. Our institution is a busy urban ED in the southeast with over 400 SCD patient visits per year. Patient satisfaction scores measured from returned surveys, verbal feedback from patients, verbal feedback from SCD outpatient providers, and physician frustration with high admission rates (i.e., failure to control pain during the ED encounter), along with changes in hospital reimbursement for admissions of SCD patients, made clear to ED leadership that an improved, evidence-based intervention for this population was needed. While many patients with SCD pain can control pain outside of the ED, other patients come to the ED more frequently as pain crises might occur at off hours and on weekends when primary care is not available. The subjective nature of this pain as well as the need for parenteral opioid utilization by many patients creates a suspicion for "drug seeking" (the EM physician term usually reserved for patients requesting or manipulating an encounter to receive parenteral opioids) as well as "frequent-flier."

"Frequent-flier" is a pejorative term that ED staff reserve for known "super-utilizers," the term used by hospital administration to define those who visit the ED multiple times in one year (chapter 7). Often these individuals have an illness that is not readily explained by biomedical models of organic disease and may also pose financial challenges to the hospital as many do not have the ability to pay for the visit, and even third-party insurers may not be willing to pay for multiple visits.

Nationally, approximately one-third of SCD-related ED visits are represented by frequent users that visit more than three times each year. The other two-thirds of patients had zero previous visits during a one-year period (Aisiku et al. 2009). SCD patients that visit the ED more than three times per year were found to have higher pain scores on both VOC and non-VOC days, potentially causing them to visit the ED more often (Aisiku et al. 2009).

The National Heart, Lung and Blood Institute publishes best practice guidelines for management of patients with SCD-related pain (NHLBI 2014). Those guidelines recommend first dose of pain medication for patients presenting to the ED within 30 minutes of arrival and the utilization of a consistent pain management delivery strategy (2014). For example, patient-controlled analgesia (PCA) is a delivery system for intravenous pain medication that can provide a bolus of analgesia, a steady-state delivery continuous infusion of medication and patient-controlled intermittent boluses of medication and predetermined safe intervals. NHLBI data demonstrate that hospital systems following best practice guidelines can reduce admission rates from the ED for sickle cell patients as well as lengths of stay (LOS) in which admission is needed. Hospital systems are financially interested in reducing SCD-related admissions as many patients with SCD have Medicaid as their primary payer. Medicaid may pay 50% to 70% of Medicare rates and significantly less than private insurance (e.g., 5% to 10% of some contracted insurance rates).

TGH ED WORK WITH SCD PATIENTS PRIOR TO WORK WITH CLINICALLY APPLIED ANTHROPOLOGISTS

Prior to 2016, EM physicians in the TGH ED provided variable care to patients that presented to the ED with sickle cell pain crisis. Pain is a subjective experience in which suffering is embodied by patients with wide variation leading to potential for individual physician biases to enter judgments of deservingness for whether a patient should or should not receive pain medication. Patients often had long lengths of stay (LOS) observed in the exceeding eight hours (goal is three hours for patients discharged home and less than four hours for patients admitted to the hospital) and, when they were admitted, had long hospital LOS as well. In addition, patient satisfaction data demonstrated that these patients felt marginalized, recognized the variability in their care plans, and were unhappy with care at our institution (but continued to come to this hospital as we are the academic center with a specialty hematologist caring for them as an outpatient that is on medical staff).

When patients with SCD are admitted to the hospital, the LOS for those patients exceeds the hospital median LOS (5.7 days). TGH ED leadership, including JWW, wanted to decrease admission rates by following NHLBI best practices including early pain management (within 30 minutes of patient arrival) and a consistent pain management strategy with low variability across providers by utilizing PCA delivery of opioid medications at standard, predetermined, dosing. In addition, we wanted to decrease SCD associated stigma related to these patient encounters in order improve the patient experience measured by patient satisfaction scores.

Specifically, we hypothesized that encounter variation led to increased LOS and high admission rates (>50% of SCD pain encounters) by implementing an NHLBI based pain management strategy. During a one-year period from May 1, 2015, to April 30, 2017, there were 1,785 SCD encounters related to pain crisis, representing 189 unique patients. On average, there are 2.25 SCD encounters and each patient of the 190 SCD patients returns approximately every 3.86 days for treatment of VOC. All encounters were reviewed creating a benchmark baseline data set for pre- and post-intervention analysis. This data was compared to post-intervention data (May 1, 2017to April 30, 2019).

We found that the number of unique patient visits increased over time, but the rate of those visits decreased from 2.25 encounters per day to 1.33 encounters per day. Each patient among the population of unique SCD patients that encountered our ED during the study period also visited less often, decreasing their visit rate by 38% (table 8.1, Osorno-Cruz and Wilson 2018).

Baseline data demonstrated that patients presenting to the TGH ED had an admission rate of 64%, compared to average hospital admission rate for all-comers to the ED of 42%. After implementation of the PCA, the admission rate declined from 64% in 2015 to 59% in 2017 among patients presenting with SCD VOC (-7.2%). In addition, the ED LOS did not increase more than the entire ED LOS increased during the same time period for all patients (18%). During the period reviewed, the rate of patients that left without being seen and against medical advice also decreased by 33%. The hospital LOS for admitted patients with SCD VOC did not change significantly during this period. The results were presented by, then resident, EM physician Alex Nappi at the American College of Emergency Physicians Scientific Assembly in 2016 (Nappi and Wilson 2016). Quantitatively, these results were considered a success driven by the PCA implementation.

However, patients that received a PCA did have a longer time until pain medication administration (47 minutes). The overall rate of PCA use increased from 8% to 65% during this period (table 8 1).

The admission rate decreased after widespread PCA use but the ED LOS did not go up and the AMA/LWOT rate decreased, suggesting a positive impact of the PCA on patient flow.

Unfortunately, following the initial launch of our NHBLI based PCA intervention, patient experiences and patient satisfaction scores among SCD patients did not improve, even though admission rates decreased and, overall, more pain medication was delivered in the ED. These findings were surprising to the ED leadership team including JWW and the team was unsure why

Table 8.1 Change in Patient Throughput Metrics after Implementation of a PCA Pain Management Strategy in SCD VOC in the ED.

Sickle Cell Patients May 1, 2015 - April 30, 2017	ALL	PCA	NO PCA	2015	2016	2017	% CHANGE 2015 - 2017
TOTAL NUMBER OF ENCOUNTERS	1635	665	969	567	814	254	
NUMBER OF UNIQUE PATIENTS	189	122	121	100	144	79	
SICKLE CELL PATIENT ENCOUNTERS PER DAY	2.25	1.10	1.33	2.32	2.23	2.08	10%
SICKLE CELL PATIENT UNIQUE VISIT RATE	0.26	0.17	0.17	0.41	0.59	0.32	-38%
SICKLE CELL PATIENT ENCOUNTERS PER 100000 PATIENTS PER DAY	2.92	1.42	1.73	0.53	0.77	0.42	21%
ADMITTED	953	383	570	361	444	150	17%
ADMIT PERCENT	58%	58%	59%	64%	55%	59%	7.2%
DISCHARGED	665	277	388	206	370	104	-0.97%
DISCHARGED PERCENT	41%	42%	40%	36%	45%	41%	11%
OTHER (AMA, LWOT)	16	5	11	9	4	3	33%
OTHER (AMA, LWOT) PERCENT	0.98%	0.75%	1.14%	1.59%	0.49%	1.18%	26%
ED LOS	6:03:00	6:03:00	6:02:00	5:55:00	5:54:00	6:57:00	18%
HOSPITAL LOS	2	2	2	3	1	2	33%
ESI SCORE	2	2	2	2	2	2	0
DOOR TO PAIN MEDICATION	37:00.0	47:00.0	30:00.0	29:00.0	37:00.0	2:04:00	28%
FIRST MEDICATION TO SECOND MEDICATION	UNKNOWN	UNKNOWN	UNKNOWN	UNKNOWN	UNKNOWN	UNKNOWN	
TREATED TO DISPO	4:13	4:11	4:16	4:08	4:12	4:24	18%
RATE OF PCA USE	40.67%	NA	NA	8%	56%	65%	53%

Source: Reproduced from Osorno-Cruz and Wilson, 2018.

patient perceptions of our intervention were different than ours and why we were falling short of patient expectations. After continuing our PCA use, our patient throughput and satisfaction data held flat, suggesting that other, unknown, important factors were limiting the team's ability to make further improvements. Flat quantitative and unclear direction creates an ideal environment for mixed methods studies using qualitative data to drive new hypotheses. We did note that there was also a plateau of using the PCA order among physicians for treating patients with SCD-related pain and wondered if implicit biases were leading to SCD VOC pain management pathway resistance among frontline ED physicians and nurses. This lukewarm pathway support may have also led to poor pathway support and communication from ED staff and physicians when talking with patients, increasing distrust.

THE ANTHROPOLOGICAL DIFFERENCE

To better understand these gaps between clinical throughput metric improvement and flattening of patient experience feedback, as well as resistance to SCD VOC pain management PCA order utilization by physicians, we conducted qualitative, semi-structured interviews with ED providers, frontline staff, hematologists, and, most importantly, patients who had SCD while in the ED. An undergraduate premedical student, Carlos Osorno (now a medical student at the University of Iowa), who had previously taken our TGH class (see chapter 3) conducted these interviews and presented preliminary results of this work at the state EM conference in Florida (Osorno-Cruz, Nappi, and

Wilson 2017) and the Society for Applied Anthropology conference (Osorno-Cruz and Wilson, 2018). The patient-generated insights allowed us to identify pathway gaps that needed improvement.

SCD PATIENT INTERVIEW RESULTS (FROM CARLOS OSORNO)

The following narratives with Marvin and Mary are from interviews conducted by Carlos Osorno-Cruz, and we have included his first-person writing contribution below.

MARVIN

My (CO) first encounter with a sickle cell patient was in the ED during one of my overnight shifts. Marvin came to the ED with complaints of a pain crisis. I was told by the attending physician (JWW) he would be a great patient to talk to about SCD and SCD pain management in the ED. The attending physician did not tell me that the patient would be defined as a super-utilizer and is well-known to hospital staff. I knocked on the door to the patient's room and I was greeted by a pleasant African American male in his mid-20s. I took a seat beside him, and we talked about his disease. He told me in lay terms what sickle cell was and that he was born with the disease. Nonchalantly he told me that he would die at an early age because of this "horrible disease." Marvin emphasized his experience in suffering, focusing on his baseline pain and how, during a crisis like the one he was suffering while we talked, the pain became uncontrollable. I asked Marvin if he had any family with SCD. He mentioned that his brother has SCD, as well as a few friends but most of them had "passed" already. He made it very clear to me that healthcare providers, family, and friends do not understand the pain that him and his brother go through. As a young boy, Marvin said he was in and out of school and the hospital frequently because of pain crises. His other siblings who only carried the Sickle Cell Trait did not have the same health issues that he and his brother have endured.

"It's very much like a man not being able to understand the pain a woman goes through during birth," Marvin said. In his case, "it doesn't matter what gender or sex you are, if you don't have sickle cell then you don't understand SCD related pain." Marvin and I continued discussing his current ED visit. I asked him, "How's your visit so far?" In a gloomy voice he said, "It's ok, I've been waiting for many hours and no one has come to see me."

Marvin felt like his care varied from time to time depending on the healthcare team that saw him on any given day but stated that he has gotten used to it. My (CO) other conversations with ED administrators echoed this reflection and the 2015 pathway was aimed at trying to decrease that variability in treatment approaches through a more uniform SCD pain management pathway.

Marvin knew the names of the doctors and nurses who he liked and disliked. He did not care if he received his pain medication through PCA or push (injection) because he just wanted his pain to be controlled as soon as possible. Although, he feels that the PCA method is giving him less pain medication than traditional delivery routes (intravenous or intramuscular push injection) because he was not receiving any when he would fall asleep (JWW notes that a basal rate is set on the pump providing continuous infusion).

Marvin explained that every time that he receives the PCA there is a problem with the equipment or there isn't one available and he must wait. Once the PCA was set up, he did say he prefers the ability to self-dose as this route allows him to not bother the nurse each time he is in more pain. In follow-up discussions between myself (CO) and JWW, Marvin's words seemed to provide important insight regarding the PCA in a patient with very resistant pain and deemed as hard to manage by the ED staff may help to bridge the gaps in improving care as it appears that the barriers to accepting PCA are logistical concerns regarding equipment and educational gaps in how the medication is delivered. This insight from Marvin is different than the commonly held notion of many ED staff I talked to that often state that the patients do not like the PCA because they do not get large push doses of opioid.

Marvin continued to tell me (CO) about his experiences at our hospital and about his sickle cell pain. From the patient perspective, he appeared to be at the facility in good faith to find pain relief. I learned from staff that this patient is labeled as "Difficult" and has a "PSAP" on the chart which is a patient-specific action plan reserved for patients perceived to be combative or resistant to physician care plans. During my interactions, the patient did not seem uncooperative but instead displayed common expressions of human suffering while in pain.

MARY

Mary also has SCD. I (CO) met Mary in the outpatient infusion clinic at our institution. She was there for a checkup with her hematologist/oncologist. In the clinic, I spoke to Mary about her experiences with SCD and what she believed the best way was to approach the patients with the disease. Mary, a mother of a healthy daughter, explained to me that because of her disease she was in pain "24/7." She fights this pain with hydration and finds any type of heat to be comforting (hot water bath, hot tea, and hot washcloths) which, Mary says, works most of the time. Occasionally, she goes into a

VOC resulting in intolerable pain leading to the use of her prescribed opioids. Mary says that she tries to take her pain medication only when needed because she understands that her tolerance to opioids will increase if she uses it daily. When her home medications do not work, she would take a trip to the ED hoping that they could handle her pain without having to admit her "to prison."

Mary like many of the other patients that I talked to did not want to be admitted from the ED to the inpatient hospital floor. Through participant observation and discussion with numerous ED physicians, it seemed as though many physicians and staff in the ED believe the opposite regarding the patient's goals during the visit. Since, historically, over 60% of patients do get admitted while in a SCD-related pain crisis, many staff members we (CO and JWW) spoke with believe this is the disposition the patient desires on arrival. For a variety of reasons, patients are admitted on average for almost six days into the hospital causing them to be absent to their jobs and families. JWW notes that the observed provider to provider variation in ED practice is multiplied exponentially in the hospital setting with multiple physician teams and nursing staff members interacting with the patient throughout the visit. If a pathway still has variability in the ED, it is unlikely that any improvement would be seen in the hospital setting as the patient moves further away from the ED order set. During a hospital admission, patients must find someone who can babysit their kids, while experiencing increased possibilities of job loss or behind in school.

Mary told me (CO) an unforgettable story about her younger sister's experience at another hospital. Her sister was going through a VOC and decided to go to the ED, seeking pain relief. At the hospital, she waited four hours before she was given any sort of treatment. Unfortunately, Mary believes that her sister's crisis was not taken seriously, and that inaction led to an avoidable coma. Mary recommends that healthcare providers ask them, "What works for you?" during triage. It's the first few minutes with the triage nurse that set the mood with the patient according to Mary. JWW notes that, at our facility, we recognize the importance of these early interactions and empower triage nurses to utilize a SCD nurse-initiated pain protocol (NIPP) which does allow for the administration of opioid medications. However, continued bias regarding perceived drug-seeking behavior among the SCD patients by ED staff led to a 0% pain medication utilization rate within the NIPP over a one-year period (2017–2018). Mary states, "We can tell if the nurse is listening or not. We know our disease better than they do."

JWW and CO discussed the hours CO had spent conducting participant observation in the ED with SCD VOC patients in the context of JWW's thousands of hours of clinical experiences and work with other physicians and nurses. JWW and CO note that sickle cell patients have experienced the excruciating pain of their disease all their lives and the use of opioids to help treat SCD-related pain creates a tolerance for high doses of opioids. When patients tell a nurse that they need 4 milligrams of hydromorphone (a potent opioid 8 to 10 times stronger than morphine) they often ignore the volume of drug requested by the patient. In some patients 4 milligrams is physiologically required secondary to pharmacodynamics of opioid pain medications in which larger and larger doses are required over time to have the same perceived impact on symptoms after the drugs block Mu receptors. There is also evidence that the earlier pain medication is administered, the more likely it is that a patient will be discharged from the ED, avoiding the "prison."

HEALTHCARE PROVIDER INTERVIEWS AND PARTICIPANT OBSERVATION BY CARLOS OSORNO-CRUZ

When I (CO) mention sickle cell patients to ED providers at our facility, the first patient that comes to mind is Marvin. A few days after speaking to Marvin I found out that during the same encounter was also his first day back from jail. On his last visit to the hospital Marvin assaulted a nurse and other healthcare professionals. I was shocked when I heard this because the person I spoke to did not seem like someone who would commit such an act so I asked myself, "What caused his frustration?"

Marvin had been in the waiting room for hours, then brought back to the exam room and still had to wait more time for his first dose of pain medication. My next question was "Why is it taking so long to administer pain medication if we have a protocol?" I thought the best person to ask would be the nurses who see these patients first and can order an initial dose of pain medication within the framework of the SCD NIPP.

The responses from multiples nurses demonstrate a widely held staff perception that SCD patients are "just drug seeking," and that "they are taking advantage of us," or "if we give them what they want they won't stop coming." The SCD patient population has been stigmatized in the ED as drug seekers just like Monica Mann describes in her story of Solomon (Mann, 2010). Solomon, an immigrant from Africa, had a VOC while traveling on a train and collapsed from the excruciating pain that it caused. Solomon could overhear spectators call him a "druggie" and "homeless guy." When he was being triaged, he told his nurse that acetaminophen would not be enough, and she told him, "Let me do my job." I (CO) recounted this story to JWW, and he stated,

> It's important to understand the difference between medically necessary and unnecessary drug seeking. When we have allergies, we seek for medication that

> will relieve those symptoms. When a patient wants medication for their own recreational pleasure then that is medically unnecessary drug seeking. Sickle cell patients who have a real disease with real symptoms seek pain medication to relieve their symptoms just like you do when you may seek caffeine when waking up in the morning suggesting that SCD patients may experience unnecessary prolonged delays in medication administration.

According to the National Institute of Health, a patient with SCD receives an initial dose of pain medication within 60 minutes of arrival to the ED (NHLBI 2014). Currently, patients at the study site ED receive the first dose of pain medications in a mean time of 90 minutes. The sooner patients receive pain medication the less likely they are to be admitted into the hospital (2014). There is an existing approved pathway to correct the long door to drug times, but this pathway (the nursing NIPP) is not utilized secondary to preconceptions from medical staff regarding patient visit motivations.

The healthcare providers view all sickle cell patients as high utilizers when only one-third of the population visit more than three times a year. When speaking to healthcare staff (nurses, techs, and some physicians) there is a widely shared belief that patients are receiving more medication through the PCA. Other institutions have demonstrated that patients receive less pain medication on the PCA compared to traditional push method in the same amount of time (Santos et al. 2015). Much of the frontline ED staff feel that setting up a PCA pump is a waste of time and contribute to the support of a patient "addiction." Staff members feel that the PCA pumps take too long to set up, mainly because parts during the initial roll out were often missing or broken. Indeed, after further investigation this was true and with the support of the hospital, the ED purchased additional PCA pumps that are used only for sickle cell patients in the department.

CONCLUSION

Our work to decrease stigma of SCD VOC and to normalize PCA pain management pathways that deliver analgesia invariably, quickly, and consistently is ongoing. While much of our quantitative data did show improvements, that data stopped moving in a positive direction. By utilizing a mixed methods approach involving participant observation and interviews, important insights surfaced. Specifically, patient misperceptions about amount of drug in the PCA are an important nidus for education. In addition, the delay in analgesia administration led to purchase of more PCA units and mandatory nurse training on their use. The variability that exists after admission and outside of the ED is also addressed through an interdisciplinary hospital team that includes JWW along with nursing leaders, social workers, hematologists, outpatient providers, hospitalists, and pain medicine experts. JWW has recently received funding to initiate new strategies to deliver analgesia more quickly through a sublingual form—specifically addressing the patient concerns that Carlos uncovered by bridging the time while the PCA is set up. Carlos's work with SCD patients at our institution also led to participation as a member site of the Alliance Quality Initiative, where our results were shared across other EDs supported by NHLBI. The increased visibility being brought to this patient population has led to some reduction of stigma and less variable practice patterns just through the un-entanglement of biases from real patient suffering and the need to continue delivering high-quality healthcare.

Our interviews and qualitative data support the utilization of PCAs and suggest that barriers to utilization that staff believe exist (i.e., the patients don't like it because they don't get a push dose and we are giving "addicts" even more pain medication) are likely not the true barriers to patient resistance to this pathway. Instead, SCD patients are concerned with fair communication and having the trust that the providers and staff are taking their pain seriously. In addition, logistical and resource supply issues seem to be the major drivers relating to negative patient feelings regarding the PCA. We hope that, ultimately, the goals of the patient may align with the goals of the ED physician—to receive a MSE, a chance to rule out an EMC, control of pain, and ultimately the best disposition for the patient which may be back home and not to the "prison."

Chapter 9

Language, Pain, and Nontraditional Patient Treatment Spaces

Contributions by Seiichi Villalona

Our work with Seiichi Villalona expanded the potential for how we could utilize graduate student anthropologists and premedical students in the clinical space since Seiichi was both during his time in the Emergency Department (ED). Seiichi spent over three years in the ED working as a research assistant (RA) for JWW and the graduate assistant for the undergraduate course taught by JWW and RBB (chapter 3). Where our undergraduate honors theses project ideas sagged (because of time and experience), we learned that a motivated graduate student (especially one that was conducting long-term participant observation through their role as an RA) could certainly enhance and push forward mixed methods projects with complicated patient populations in acute clinical spaces. Seiichi's experiences, first taking the undergraduate class, serving as the graduate assistant for the class, working in the ED, and desire to go to medical school crafted an ideal scenario where he was able to understand some of the questions relevant clinically and to patients—a gap that is hard to fit into without an approach like ours. While Seiichi went to medical school, we envision a role that a graduate student could continue as a career in patient experience after the type of work that Seiichi did during the completion of his MA thesis.

This chapter discusses a medical anthropology approach to patient experience and patient satisfaction. Villalona utilized an existing data set (six years of patient satisfaction surveys) to explore craft hypotheses regarding patients with limited English proficiency (LEP), patients placed into nontraditional care spaces (e.g., hallways), and patients that were in pain. Seiichi used this existing data (both quantitative and qualitative) to craft hypotheses that he tested in the ED through participant observation and patient interviews. This work led to confirmation that many patient challenges (language, hallways pain) can be overcome when communication between the healthcare staff and the patient is emphasized (see chapter 6). This chapter covers the background and context that drove Seiichi's work and provides an overview of those findings.

BACKGROUND

Modern biomedicine translates patient-centered care and patient experiences into the scores that providers, nurses, and hospitals receive on Hospital Consumer Assessment of Healthcare Providers (HCAHP, n.d.) surveys. These surveys are often administered by Press-Ganey (Press-Ganey Associates n.d.). While they are replete with all the problems of surveys data collection, they are the language of experience in the current healthcare environment. Thus, to engage providers and healthcare systems in patient-centered care and improvements to the patient experience, the frame must be around improvements into Press-Ganey survey scores to obtain buy-in for potential interventions and meaningfulness of observational qualitative and analysis of quantitative data. We developed a series of mixed methods projects with Seiichi that sought to identify areas for improvement in patient satisfaction scores specifically when considering patients with LEP, patients placed into non-approved or nontraditional patient care spaces (e.g., the hallway), and patients that may have been upset with the ED encounter secondary to the perceived dismissal or lack of adequate pain management.

We hypothesize that the ceiling for improvement of patient satisfaction scores is limited with a narrow range for potential interventions to lead to increases in scores. This limitation is secondary to the decisions of deservingness around patient care selection and the development of patient pathways. Patients with structured, predetermined, essentialist categories of emergency medical conditions (stroke, heart attack, blood stream infection with low blood pressure, a new infectious disease spreading across the globe) are visualized by care providers and healthcare systems, extracted from the heaps of reality in the ED waiting room. Those patients left behind may not turn as many surveys, or, perhaps, they are unable to complete the survey, or do not have an easy way to turn the survey back in (language, homelessness, reading level).

Who are those patients? Those are special populations potentially seen to add only cost to the revenue margins or difficulty to the preferred strictly medical care pathway. We have recognized patients with Sickle Cell Disease (SCD), firearm violence, and opioid use disorder as specific groups of patients and we discuss their care more in chapters 8, 11, and 10. Patients with LEP may receive surveys that they cannot answer or express the frustrations of the everyday violence those patients might undergo when their 10-year-old children are asked to interpret for them about issues of a diagnosis of vaginal discharge, a sexual history, or sensitive histories of HIV, IV drug use, or sex work. LEP patients are a special population that, given current variation in approach, may perpetuate low scores on patient experience surveys.

Not all patients who enter the ED ever make it into a private bed. This may be an acceptable expectation in some parts of the world, but in the United States, the modern hospital is associated with the luxury of private room and private space. Revenue pressures facing hospitals lead to open beds on floors (room for elective surgical patients with predictable reimbursements) while ED patients may remain in the ED for hours after a hospital admission, driving waiting room lines longer and waiting room crowds larger. Hospital EDs across the United States are left to deal with these boarding pressures through "front-end processes"—which essentially means a recognition that the admission process is unlikely to change in the current healthcare delivery climate and, thus, the ED staff need to make do, enhance, and creatively interpret the space that they do have left. During the aftermath of Covid-19, staffing shortages for environmental service workers, patient care technicians, and even nurses have combined with the already problematic revenue models (e.g., emphasis on prioritizing beds for elective surgery patients over ED patients that are admitted to the hospital given the predictable, and potentially higher, revenue stream) that lead to open floor beds to synergize and worsen the problem of ED crowding. Wein and Wilson (2009) demonstrated that when 10% of total available bed hours (e.g., numbers of approved bed spaces in the ED multiplied by the number of hours each day those beds are operational) are taken up by boarded patients (patients admitted to the hospital but still in the ED), other patient experience and patient safety metrics begin to worsen exponentially (e.g., waiting room times to see a physician and the number of people who grow frustrated at these long waits and then leave the ED without being seen). After the peak of Covid-19, beginning in the spring of 2021, hospital EDs began to boarding times that are 10 times worse than what was observed in 2009 data. Some EDs are now dealing with 100% or more of available beds occupied by admitted patients with admission rates that have not changed for over a decade (JWW personal communication with other NIH ED Principal Investigators and other medical directors throughout the United States in May and June 2021). Where do we place patients instead? For a long time now, there has been a realization that boarding is a feature of modern healthcare delivery. EDs have created treatment spaces, referred to as non-approved or nontraditional patient care spaces; these spaces are often a gurney or chair in the hallway (or sometimes a recliner chair in the waiting room). Patients might remain in that space for the bulk of their ED stay. How does nontraditional patient care space (e.g., hallways) affect the overall ED encounter and experience?

Many providers are distrustful of Press-Ganey patient survey data (Jones 2018, Birdstrike et al. 2013). Overall, few patients return the surveys. What is the motivation for the patients that do return the surveys? Irwin Press (2006) and Dempsey (2017) have demonstrated that, over time, the sample size of surveys for a single provider (or healthcare system) becomes sufficient and the low response rate eventually becomes less important as that sample size increases. But do only angry patients return the surveys? No—there is no data to support this. However, the myth that patients become angry and use the survey to tell off doctors is perpetuated in medicine. The myth is furthered by the assumption that the angry patient is likely a "drug seeker" who wants IV opioid pain medications or a prescription for strong oral pain medications, does not get those medications, and then turns in an angry, negative survey. While this is not supported by the data, the surveys were changed to ask less about how pain was specifically controlled during an acute encounter and instead to ask if pain was discussed during the acute encounter (Hoffman et al. 2016). Whether deemed legitimate and deserving by care providers (e.g., cancer patients with terminal disease) or non-deserving (e.g., regional pain syndrome, chronic pain, SCD pain crisis), pain and associated suffering do occupy much of the care negotiation space between patients and physicians.

METHODS

Villalona utilized a mixed methods approach (both qualitative and quantitative, as well as retrospective and prospective) that considered the potential impacts on patient experience and patient satisfaction during ED encounters among LEP patients, patients placed in hallways, and patients that mentioned pain management as a concern. This work specifically utilized 6 years of deidentified ED Press-Ganey survey data available to our institution from January 1, 2012, to January 31, 2017, representing over 4,000 patient encounters. Those data included both numerical responses to survey questions and patient provided comments to open-ended questions at the end of the survey. In addition to analysis of retrospective survey data, Seiichi spent over 2,500 hours in the ED, specifically observed 100 LEP physician-patient encounters, and conducted semi-structured interviews with 25 patients in Spanish. As Seiichi progressed through his graduate school education, he continued to utilize the provided Press-Ganey data set, considering enhanced ways to conduct analysis and new variations of questions to pose retrospectively and prospectively as his skill set (e.g., biostatistics, anthropological methods) and knowledge base (what matters to Emergency Medicine [EM] physicians, administrators, and patients) progressed in parallel.

LEP

Most patients in the United States who enter the ED are fluent, native English speakers, and most of the patients who return patient satisfaction surveys measuring their patient experience are fluent, native English speakers. But even when both the patient and physician are fluent native English speakers, there are many opportunities to improve patient satisfaction scores related to consistent themes of communication gaps between physicians, other healthcare staff, and patients. The exploration of illness and structural determinants of suffering are limited even when the patient and the physician both speak fluent, native English. Imagine just how much worse these healthcare encounters are when a patient speaks no or limited English—or, worse yet, when a non-English-speaking patient is also placed in nonstandard care space secondary to hospital overcrowding (e.g., a hallway chair).

Patients with limited English proficiency (LEP) suffer more medical errors (Flores et al. 2012) and have more difficulty with follow-up plans (Silva et al. 2014). Essentially, those patients under-experience care and the limited experiences they do have are hidden by lack of adequate data collection bearing witness. LEP may also represent a form of structural violence as patients seek care in clinical spaces in which they do not know whether there will be adequate open access to professional interpreters that speak their native language. LEP is an ideal space for an applied medical anthropologist to make contributions—there is a socially mediated determinant that has an impact on a specific medical outcome (Jacobs et al. 2019 demonstrated that LEP patients have higher sepsis mortality), a worse patient experience, and, secondary to low patient satisfaction scores and disparities in health outcomes, may impact provider and institution reimbursement.

There are three important ongoing issues with LEP patients: (1) Is there continuous access to a professional interpreter during a clinical encounter? (2) What is the best type of interpreter modality to use for patients (i.e., phone, video, live professional interpreter, live ad hoc family member, or staff)? (3) Is the available modality used during the entire clinical encounter (i.e., just because the physician and patient have access to the interpreter, are they using the interpreter)? In this chapter, we outline work we have done with students to first observe and analyze the experiences of LEP patients in our ED and then to test specific interpreter modalities while finding ways to implement their usage. Much of this work was done with Seiichi Villalona who worked in the ED as a RA with a focus on language-related patient experiences. Seiichi completed his MA thesis based on his work examining patient-physician interactions limited by LEP among Spanish speaking patients (Villalona 2018). Seiichi is now a medical student at the Rutgers Robert Wood Johnson Medical School. His graduate work in applied medical anthropology embodies our focus to intervene early in the training of future physicians, preparing them to view their work through the lens of patient experience. Seiichi's passion for LEP was contagious and drew interest of one of the prior EM residents, Christian Jeanot, who grew up in Florida but was originally from Haiti. Christian speaks fluent Creole and most of our student and resident-led work on LEP has been with Spanish speaking and Creole speaking patients at the Tampa General Hospital (TGH) ED. In addition, Mary Yanez Yuncosa was a prior undergraduate student who took our ED-based patient-physician interaction course and remained active in the ED as a RA, later completing her undergraduate honors thesis examining issues of LEP in the ED. Mary Yunez Yucosa worked with myself (JWW), Villalona, and Christian Jeanot on much of the data collected and presented in this chapter outlining how applied medical anthropologists can identify and work to improve healthcare delivery barriers related to LEP as well as how physicians and physicians in training can emphasize the removal of LEP barriers in their everyday clinical encounters. The model of a graduate student, premedical student, and resident physician working together on a patient-centered mixed methods project was also important for us to adopt and scale across other projects.

Villalona et al., 2019 demonstrated that, even when interpretation devices are available, the use of interpretation services is highly variable across patient encounters in the ED and clinical space (Crossman et al. 2010, Diamond et al. 2009, Lopez et al. 2015, Mayo et al. 2016). This variability is secondary to provider preferences (some providers are more likely to use interpretation services than others), ease of use (how quickly and readily available is the interpretation service) as well as timing and number of interactions during the encounter. In other words, maybe the physician uses the interpretation phone service to gather the history and initial physical exam (H&P) from the patient but does not use the phone service on subsequent encounters. One likely scenario in the ED is that nurse and physician both use an interpreter service initially but when an emergent disease state is ruled out, those same healthcare team members do not use the phone service again to explain possible explanations or treatment pathways for the illness (which they may determine is less important to communicate than the steps to take in the setting of disease).

In the United States, 27 million people speak Spanish as their primary language (Krogstad et al. 2015). Our work in Florida, a state with a higher representation of Spanish speakers, is situated in Hillsborough County where there are almost 300,000 people who speak Spanish as their first language. In addition, Spanish speaking patients are more likely to have limited access to primary care and more likely to access the ED (Florida DOH 2017).

Our team wanted to know more about how physician utilization of interpretation services affected patient experiences in the ED and designed a cross-sectional study to examine the impact (Villalona et al. 2019). Seiichi and Mary are native Spanish speakers. Each of those students approached and consented 100 Spanish-speaking patients early in their ED course (right after triage) and observed those patients again at the end of the ED visit. In a novel approach to gathering patient feedback, Seiichi led the team (Villalona et al. 2020) of students to conduct a modified version of the standard Press-Ganey Hospital Consumer Assessment of Healthcare Providers and Systems (HCAHPS 2021) survey along with a Visual Analog Scale (VAS) to obtain a single point measurement of patient satisfaction with the visit (highly satisfied to highly dissatisfied). Higher VAS scores represented higher satisfaction. The team broke down survey responses by the type of interpretation service that was used (no interpretation, ad hoc family member or staff, phone, or video) and compared satisfaction scores among each group using a nonparametric statistical test (Kruskal-Wallis). The group of patients that received professional interpretation services of any kind outperformed those that did not and had the highest patient satisfaction scores. In addition, those patients that received a video interpretation service had both the highest VAS scores and the least variability between patients in that group. Interestingly though, while video outperformed every category at every stage of the visit (post triage and time of discharge) use of ED staff that spoke Spanish outperformed phone interpretation at discharge. In other words, it appears that patients appreciate a human touch to discussions surrounding follow-up plans and a visually enhanced interaction is preferred.

Hundred Spanish speaking patients received the patient satisfaction survey. A 25-sample subset of those patients also underwent semi-structured interviews in Spanish with either Seiichi or Mary regarding their experiences and their survey answers. Interviews were coded and thematic analysis was conducted. This qualitative interview analysis complements our quantitative survey results, providing a window into the drivers of why some LEP patients have a poor experience and what can be done to improve overall satisfaction.

There were three themes that stood out among the 25 patient interviews: (1) Limitations to patient autonomy, (2) Lack of clarity in follow-up plans, and (3) Feelings of self-blame (for having LEP). Issues of autonomy were detailed by nine participants who emphasized how important having professional interpretation services were at every visit to facilitate communication with staff and explain to staff, in their own words, their current medical problem and past medical history. Twelve patients felt that the use of interpretation services was necessary to ensure understanding of why diagnostic tests were being done, test results, and ability to ask the staff questions and to receive detailed information regarding follow-up care plans. Five of the patients feared a potential miscommunication or error in the absence of interpretation services.

LEP also limits autonomy—part of the patient experience during the clinical encounter is to tell a story. Patients place emphasis on their own story and the construction of a narrative that connects their illness to possible disease, allowing the healthcare team access into the cognitive underpinnings of the patient's embodiment of their own chief complaint. However, LEP patients have difficulty in expressing their narrative and feel that the most controllable part of their healthcare encounter is limited by this inability to craft a story of their visit. In addition, Seiichi and the team have demonstrated that this lack of autonomy is magnified after the initial encounter between the patient and the healthcare team. That initial encounter may consist of a provider utilizing professional interpretation services, but after this data is collected, hours may go by before an interpreter is again utilized. The extract contains quotes from patient interviews that emphasize the impact on autonomy and the structural violence and power differentials associated with LEP and patient self-blame for not being native fluent English speakers.:

> It feels frustrating and it would be better if I could speak directly to staff because I could say exactly what I need to say.
>
> After they ask you the question in the beginning you just sit here and wait. You worry more when you can't understand what is happening.
>
> They come in and tell you something quickly and you say "OK" and then you try to figure out what they are really telling you.
>
> Maybe I need to learn English instead since we are in a country where the main language is English. It makes it a lot easier to be able to tell them exactly what symptoms you are feeling.
>
> I can't complain. They do their best to help, even if they can't understand me. It's us that have to do a better job at understanding them by learning English.
>
> We are very happy with any help they can provide. We understand that this is not our country and that Spanish is not what everyone speaks.
>
> It is not their fault that they do not understand us, we should understand them. I know they do the best they can, although it's really hard for me to understand them.

Villalona surveyed patients using a Spanish version of the Press-Ganey evaluation tool that was currently being mailed to patients after an ED visit. In our modified delivery of this survey, the questions were asked in Spanish at the end of the patient encounter. This allowed for immediate feedback but is a methodological deviation from the way in which regular ED surveys are delivered outside of this project—they are mailed out over the next couple of weeks. Thus, our data may be impacted by the more immediate nature of the patient responses. However, very few Spanish speaking patients return surveys, thus, we felt that any data from an LEP sample was better than no data at all.

Overall, the survey results demonstrate that LEP has a negative impact on patient experiences in the ED (Villalona 2018, 2020a, 2020c). Overall, our goal is for patient responses to be at the "Always" level over 85% of the time. As survey responses fall below that 85% threshold, the comparison of your hospital or you as a provider (survey results can be stratified both ways) to a group of other hospitals or peers will drop in very quartiles very rapidly. In other words, the spread around the mean of survey results across institutions or providers is very narrow and the drop-off outside of that spread is drastic. This was once discussed in relation to a comparison of the Olympic sprinter Usain Bolt with other sprinters. At the time of this writing, Usain Bolt holds the world record for the fastest 100-meter dash at 9.58 seconds. During the Rio Olympics in 2016, Bolt ran that race in 9.81 seconds, while other top runners clocked in at 9.89 seconds (Justin Gatlin, second place), and 9.91 seconds (Andre De Grasse, third place). If you ran the race in over 10 seconds, you were going to fall to at least 7th place and if you dropped to over 11 seconds you become one of the millions of competitive high school athletes. In other words, levels of variance around excellence are tight. As institutions try to improve the patient experience measured through patient satisfaction, the mean shifts, and the standard deviation becomes narrower over time. Losing LEP surveys is a loss of data; however, that loss of data, from an operational level, is not emphasized because reentry of that data into the overall survey results would likely move down the institution and provider scores. For example, led by Seiichi and his team, we found that only 69% of LEP patients felt that the nurse demonstrated caring about their needs, only 53% felt informed throughout their visit, and only 58% felt that their concerns were taken seriously (Villalona et al. 2018, 2019). Evaluations of physicians were marginally better but would still result in a decline in satisfaction survey results, leading to a drop in the benchmark percentile of most institutions. While 83% of the surveyed LEP patients felt that the physician evaluating them paid attention to their needs, only 69% felt that the physician showed concern while providing treatment and only 76% felt that the physician took their concerns seriously (2018). Consistent with a language barrier, 51% of the LEP patients surveyed felt uninformed or under-informed by the healthcare team. As mentioned previously, a VAS was used as an overall measure of patient satisfaction at their time of disposition. VAS responses were then stratified by patient experience variables utilizing regression analysis. VAS scores strongly correlated with survey answers related to the perception of how much time nurses spent with the patient ($r = 0.71$, $p < 0.01$) and how informed patients were during their ED visit ($r = 0.73$, $p < 0.001$). Spanish language satisfaction surveys ($n = 100$) and semi-structured interviews ($n = 25$) with LEP patients suggest that these patients place a high level of importance on being actively involved in all aspects of ED care and exercising individual patient autonomy. LEP patients were anxious and concerned that their language limited their ability to thoroughly describe the illness and presenting complaint to the ED care team. In addition, LEP patients were at times dehumanized for the sake of convenience, representing another form of everyday structural violence (Villalona et al. 2018).

For example, in one scenario, a 31-year-old woman presented with a gynecological complain and her elementary school–aged son was used as a medical interpreter. Interestingly, prior studies (Engel et al. 2012) have shown that while there are clear opportunities for improved language interpretation in the ED, most LEP patients utilize the ED more than they utilize outpatient services, seemingly secondary to a trust that some form of language interpretation will be available.

The applied medical anthropology research project conducted by Villalona, Yucosa, and Jeanot and the team had an immediate and a direct impact on our ED. Previously in the ED, professional interpretation services were only offered through "the blue phone." The blue phone is a landline telephone with two receivers—one for the patient and one for the provider. The phones are supplied by a language interpretation company (Cyracom Inc, Tuscon, Arizona 2016) and are used to access a trained medical translator at any time. At the time of Seiichi's study on interpretation modalities and patient satisfaction, we only had access to video interpretation services through one computer equipped with a camera and special software. The results of Seiichi's work were so overwhelmingly positive that we have now shifted to emphasis of a Cyracom smartphone application that includes an option for a video interpretation service (figure 9.1). There is still high variability in consistent use of interpretation services across ED providers and patient encounters, as well as variation along the course of the ED visit. The need to login repeatedly to the Cyracom application and wait, even for 30 seconds, for a translator to be available is not a negligible deterrent during a busy ED shift.

The approaches we utilized with Seiichi's work introduced new ways of knowing how to study and improve patient experiences. Seiichi was able to implement a version of participant observation reminiscent of Geertz's deep hanging out (Geertz 1998) as he worked as a clinical trials RA in our ED, becoming comfortable with physician-patient-staff interactions, ED workflow, and talking with patients and providers. This knowledge allowed

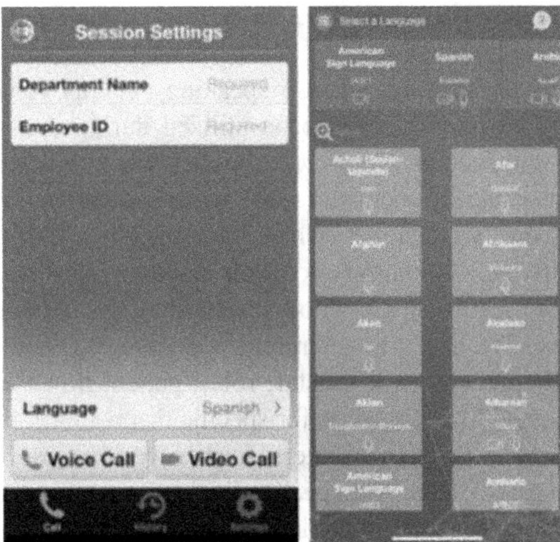

Figure 9.1 Mobile Phone Cyracom Interpreter Application. *Source*: Cyracom.com.

Seiichi to frame questions relevant to current ED work environment with answers that had applied focus and ability to close important care gaps in deservingness of those seeking care. In addition, JWW was able to provide Seiichi access to six years of data in the Press-Ganey database. This data set, all deidentified TGH ED–based patient satisfaction data, allowed for novel methodological approaches of both retrospective and prospective, quantitative, and qualitative analysis of prior 4,940 prior patient experiences (January 1, 2012, to December 31, 2017).

In Seiichi's thesis work, discussed earlier, prospective interviews and observations were completed with 100 Spanish speaking patients. However, a series of three publications also resulted from this time that combined thematic analysis of patient comments with the observational data collected during his time as a RA and completion of a master's thesis in applied anthropology. This approach was truly mixed methods as the large sample of survey questions, and standard variable responses also allowed the use of traditional parametric statistical analysis (e.g., multilinear regression) to help quantitatively test qualitative hypotheses. For example, we hypothesized that patients in pain or seeking pain medication might have led to lower patient satisfaction scores. Interestingly, 90% of patients in the database did not mention pain management as a concern, but, of those that did, the mention of pain management was strongly predictive of negative patient satisfaction scores (2020a, 2020b, 2020c).

We also predicted that patients placed in nontraditional care spaces (e.g., ED hallways) would have worse patient experiences than those placed in regular ED rooms. Interestingly, not only was this demonstrated quantitatively

(OR Negative Score 4.89, 95% CI: 2.96–8.05), but also qualitatively in the review of patient comments.

In Seiichi's master's thesis, Spanish speaking patients voiced a desire for consistent interpretation platforms to be utilized during their encounter. All areas of patient satisfaction scores were higher when a consistent modality (e.g., phone, video, family member, staff) was used throughout the ED care encounter. The scores were highest when, interestingly, a staff or family members were used (which is contrary to some popular ideas about appropriate interpreter selection), consistently good when video was used, and lowest with the use of a phone. The use of an interpreter was noted to be most important in understanding ED procedures (e.g., staff roles, patient flows, identification of physician, turnaround times, reasons for specific disposition). In both Seiichi's master's thesis among Spanish speakers, further work retrospectively reviewing Press-Ganey survey data, and specifically focusing on patients placed in a hallway bed, care issues (e.g., nontraditional placement, LEP, pain) were magnified when the patient felt that they did not understand what was expected to happen in the ED or what was happening during the encounter.

Overall, lack of understanding the process in the ED (UEDP) is the most predictive feature of a poor patient experience, regardless of LEP, hallway placement, or pain (UEDP OR 21.68, 95% CI: 6.89–68.2). This finding reinforces our hypothesis outlined in chapter 6 (the patient leaflet) that patient-informed communication regarding the ED process could dramatically improve the patient experience.

THE ANTHROPOLOGICAL DIFFERENCE

This chapter demonstrates both direct engagement of a medical anthropologist into a clinical space and an early intervention into the training of a premedical student to shift the clinical gaze and generate a patient-centered future physician through the praxis of anthropological research. The engagement in the clinical space utilized an applied approach to address a gap in care that impacts patient experiences and, potentially, patient outcomes and medical errors. Structural violence is inclusive of the demand that others are not offered equitable communication arrangements when care seeking (e.g., LEP), have pain dismissed as non-deserving, or are placed in nontraditional care spaces with less communication during the ED encounter. This applied work provides practical demonstration—an MA thesis (Villalona 2018) and three publications (Villalona et al. 2020a, 2020b, 2020c)—as to specifically how a mixed methods approach and the lens of an anthropologist can be inserted directly into the clinical space to improve care. In addition, at the time of this writing, Seiichi is completing his final year of medical school. The long process of "deep hanging out", patient shadowing, participant observation, roots in anthropology and direct patient interviews early in training are likely to profoundly alter the clinical gaze to remain patient-centered throughout his career.

Illustrative Quotes from Patients Receiving Care in ED Hallway Beds (Villalona et al. 2020, 2743):

ASSESSMENT OF NURSES

I was in the hallway the entire time that I was being treated. I do understand that the ER was very busy and I am appreciative that I was seen and treated but I felt invisible most of the time that I was being treated even though I was visible to everyone that walked past. I did not even have a screen up around me and at one point the screen beside my gurney was taken to use for someone else. I do not think I would have minded so much if I would have been asked if I wanted it to be used for me first.

Laying in hallway for 3 hours by nurses' station I was ignored by nurses and when ask a question they were not friendly.

From the time I got back to the hallway gurney, I was pretty much forgotten! Other than the "active diuretic" stool sample and blood—that was it! For the next 12 hours! Non-existent.

Was out in a hallway talking about my issue on a bed with a blanket and no pillow; very uncomfortable and embarrassing to have everyone walking by you listening and looking.

Since I was in a hallway it was extremely difficult to get the privacy I needed to talk to the nurses. Nurses changed shift around 6am and we couldn't find any one to help us get answers for over 2 hours.

ASSESSMENT OF DOCTORS

I brought in documentation from a test I had previously done in reference to the condition I was being seen for. Instead of moving forward with a different treatment or test, they repeated the same test I already had done to rule out a cause for ailment. They didn't check for infection, had me urinate and left it there without checking it, and did no further exams. I feel like it was a complete waste of my time to have come. I left without any indication as to what is going on.

The doctor I was admitted to was a woman and took the time to listen. The shift changed and my discharging MD was abrupt, cold, didn't have much explanation.

Dr. only came and asked me one question, never came back for results, never spent time at all, just two minutes to ask a question and my pain medication was given to me late and hours after one or two hours before the discharge.

Both doctors I saw barely spent 2 minutes in the room. They didn't express any concern for the amount of pain I was in and looked at me as if I wasn't a person. They also kept asking questions they should have had access to being that I came there by ambulance from an urgent care center.

I have many autoimmune disorders and am quite a complicated case. Once I got back in the ER, I saw many MDs—some listened, some did not—many were rushed. I felt like they dismissed my symptoms and pain since I came in with PMHx [*sic*] of various diagnoses—such as Chron's, endometriosis, celiac disease, RA [*sic*], and juvenile DM x 30 years [*sic*]. I was still in horrible pain and quite ill—thought I now with all of my medical issues, I will have pain and sickness—I obviously came to the ER because I felt something was really wrong. Just because I already had PMHx [*sic*] of these things doesn't mean that my symptoms should have been excused. It made me feel badly to be honest.

Issues were not completely examined. I had multiple issues—stomach, pains, back pains, and developing swelling and irritation of the left leg. Left leg was swelling and increasingly sensitive to touch. Issues seemed to be ignored after very (to me) cursory exam.

ASSESSMENT OF OVERALL ED EXPERIENCE

I was placed in gurney in the hallway. Staff and visitors would bump into my bed and the make-shift curtains. Conversations from the nursing station and from other rooms could be heard.

I received good medical care but the wait time and the lack of privacy due to being in the hallway is why I am rating the experience as poor.

Even though my experience wasn't the best, a lot of my irritation was in lack of privacy and communication.

Total time in the ED was approximately 8–9 hours, and the visible traffic was very low. I know that doesn't always mean much, but I was in the hallway the entire visit which was unacceptable.

Chapter 10

Opioids and Infectious Disease

Contributions by Heather Henderson

Our multiyear, multifaceted, Emergency Department (ED)-based work on opioid use disorder and infectious disease is our most formal and robust deployment of applied medical anthropologists into the clinical space to date. This work is not dictated by biomedicine but, instead, engaged in a two-way feedback system in which medical anthropological theory and methods are advanced and utilized directly in a way that develops not only clinical patient care but also anthropological theory itself. Specifically, MA thesis level research around stigma (Henderson 2018) and PhD dissertation work on learned helplessness (HH) have been combined with approaches to syndemics (Singer et al. 2003) and assemblage theory (Tsing 2017) in order to advance a new pathway for the management of patients with opioid use disorder and the treatment of hepatitis C viral infection (JWW and HH).

MEDICAL ANTHROPOLOGY AND CLINICAL PATHWAY DEVELOPMENT

ED patient care pathways are coordinated and multilayered management approaches to specific diagnoses. For example, a STEMI (acute heart attack) pathway begins with the development of prehospital care, designating expectations and best practices for hospital design (e.g., having a cardiac catheterization laboratory and an on-call interventional cardiologist), the prehospital space (e.g., 911 systems and coordinated EMS care to deliver patients to chest pain STEMI receiving facilities while receiving protocolized medications and treatments en route), to the arrival in the ED (including physician assessments, specific medications, and ED actions), to the cath lab (with best practices designed around percutaneous intervention and treatment of arterial occlusion), to the post-procedure management in the hospital (in-hospital physical therapy and medication management), and into the transition of care outside of the hospital after discharge (e.g., cardiac rehabilitation, cardiology physician appointments, specific medications). All of these pathway points may have expected process, throughput, and outcome metrics (idealized best practices that should be in protocols and specific time points that should be met during the pathway course).

ED patient care pathway development—especially for unseen and vulnerable populations—can improve healthcare outcomes, structural inequalities, and health inequities. Extending the work of Nading (2019), Tsing (2017), and Singer (2009), our work is moving medical management past static treatment options that leave some patients behind while also contributing to entanglement, assemblage, and syndemic theory

We draw on Nading (2019) to better understand the entanglements represented by patient complaints during each ED encounter. Nading, who spent time with public health frontline workers in Nicaragua, traced the attempts to prevent mosquito-borne disease. Those workers brought their own histories and politics to homes of neighbors, who also had their own histories and politics, during inspections for the standing water that perpetuates mosquito breeding. Nading found that the way those workers were deployed (e.g., who was hired, which neighborhood and homes were inspected, how the inspections were done) was entangled in the physical and historical structure of the Nicaraguan government. Real and idealized conflicts between Sandinistas and other factions also informed how data was recorded and presented. These entanglements—"the unfolding, often incidental attachments and affinities, antagonisms and animosities that bring people, nonhuman animals [and bacteria, viruses, pathogens], and things into each other's worlds . . . [entanglement] is at once a material, temporal and spatial condition" (Nading 2019:11)—are where extraction occurs, arising from the entanglements and rendering some disease and illness (and thus people) visible while other potential pathologies are left unseen, reifying the articulation of inequity and structural histories.

Recognition of entanglements extends and advances Kleinman's explanatory models of disease and illness (Kleinman et al. 1978). It is not just that the patient has a different mental model of their symptoms but what is also necessary to consider is the insight and positionality of the patient, the care provider, care pathway, and healthcare system's overall entanglement, asking to be brought to forefront during each encounter.

Tsing has described the concept of assemblages (deep network connections of humans, nonhumans, living and nonliving entities that extend the idea of an ecological web) (2017). Her work focuses on the complex global market for matsutake mushrooms and the workers who pick those mushrooms on the forest floor. Healthcare systems—hospitals, EDs, physician offices, diagnostic testing centers, laboratories, and other care spaces—represent an assemblage. The current biomedical model of healthcare, framed in a neoliberal capitalism, makes possible extraction of some assemblage elements, leaving other elements fully entangled. Medical education and the economic models of biomedicine reify each other to reproduce this salvage capitalism by enforcing and emphasizing training and recognition of disease states with clear-cut ICD codes that translate to procedural based revenues: medicine's version of supply chain capitalism (Tsing 2009). Acknowledgment of these assemblages allows for new modes of patient-centered care delivery. Tsing's assemblage theory and Nading's ideas of entanglement can be linked to consider how the entanglements of disease and illness present among the distributed assemblages of biomedical systems.

Which patients are rendered visible (heart attack, stroke, renal failure, sepsis) versus invisible (opioid withdrawal) is largely decided by which patients have clinical treatment pathways. Treatment pathways assemble for diseases that generate clinical revenue or can be extracted to improve quality metrics (which themselves are linked to facility payments). The extractive capitalism approach to care pathway development leads to a patchiness across patients in the ED that reifies and reproduces structural inequality hundreds of times a day as some disease, illness, and suffering is rewarded by a priori developed pathways and ICD-10 codes, but others remain entangled and unseen (Tsing 2017). This "patchiness" in clinical care makes room for anthropologists to consider how people, disease, and illnesses are entangled: entanglements of humans and pathogens, humans and histories, pathogens and histories (Nading 2019).

Modern biomedicine creates care pathways through processes of extractive capitalism—assigning superficial ICD-10 codes to complex underlying assemblages. Our approach envisions how medical anthropologists can utilize patient-centered approaches to the entanglements to create new assemblages that represent new treatment pathways (Nading 2019, Tsing 2015). Patients move through the ED space with their own histories, with stories that may match expected, constructed, "deserving," pathological frames and pathways or remain entangled and rendered non-visible during a care encounter (Villalona et al. 2020). This process elevates certain patients into normative categories of biomedicine, while simultaneously widening structural inequities among invisible patients, where human experiences and phenomena become patient encounters and illness narratives (e.g., "pain pill seekers") through unequal negotiations with healthcare at a given moment in time (Kleinman 1989; Roscoe, Eisenberg, and Forde 2016). This notion of deservingness of care acts as a staunch reinforcer of inequity, which eventually feeds back and reinforces medical education, initiating the same cycle again and again.

This feedback loop, generated by the intersection of state biopolitics, racism, structural violence, lived experiences (doctors and patients), and expectations (again, doctors and patients), hints at the potentiality of medical anthropology and biomedicine cocreating care that encompasses other ways of being, knowing, and treating what and who is not yet visible (Tsing 2017; Nading 2019).

EMERGENCY MEDICINE AND HIV/AIDS—ASSEMBLING ENTANGLED HISTORIES

Emergency Medicine (EM) was a nascent specialty at the peak of the HIV/AIDS crisis of the 1980s. The first board certification examination in EM was offered in 1980 (Thomas 2013) and, in 1986, there were only 67 residency training programs (there are now over 200). To ensure new specialty survival, attention was placed on ways to establish expertise in management of known and existing disease states—specifically the emergency care of all specialties. Prior to this, in the United States, the emergency "room" was a space in a hospital where newly graduated medical students would rotate through to gain experience early in their postgraduate training. There was a growing recognition that inexperienced physicians were least qualified to take care of the critically ill, especially regarding undiagnosed patients. In addition, many physicians in training did not feel comfortable with the chaotic arrival patterns during ER shifts in the setting of unpredictable patient types (e.g., a pregnant woman, an injured child, a cancer patient, a severe bone fracture). During the thick of the HIV/AIDS crisis in the mid-1980s, EM was focused on establishing billing, scope of practice, new hospital contracts, and training programs. As the discipline matured in the 1990s, the complexities of HIV screening, linkage, and treatment continued to leave the disease state outside of the domain of EM.

Eventually, EM matured into a large pivot space between multiple dispositions—inpatient hospitalization, observation status, critical care management or emergency operative, or procedural-based care. The "room" had become a department full of ancillary support staff, including nursing, paramedics, patient care technicians, radiology diagnostic modalities (X-ray, CT, MRI, ultrasound), and laboratory services. These diagnostics and support services were built to extract the revenue-generating disease from entangled webs of patients strewn about the ED waiting room. However, by the mid-2010s, a sea change began to brew. Pines et al. (2016) considered the ED, not just as a room, not just as a space limited to ruling out emergent medical conditions, but, instead, as a site that had become the pivot point of the American healthcare system.

During this time, HIV as a disease was largely ignored in the ED. Prior to 2015, in Florida (as with many other states), HIV testing required written patient consent, counseling before testing, and counseling after testing. In addition, before Ryan White funding, rapid linkage to care for newly diagnosed HIV could be difficult. Additionally, before 1997 and the advent of anti-retroviral therapy (ART) medications, even if HIV were to be diagnosed in the ED, treatment options were minimal. After 1997, the decision to start ART, and which ART to choose, required consultation with a specialist infectious disease physician, and patients routinely did not make or attend this appointment after a new diagnosis. Thus, the emergency physician continued to provide "supportive care" around disease states related to early HIV (e.g., sore throat, pneumonia, and skin infections) and to examine patients for known AIDS defining illness that might require hospital admission.

Beyond these routine tasks, no clear path was built for these patients that included HIV screening and linkage to treatment if positive. In 2006, however, there was a significant disruption to the nonexistent HIV screening available in the ED. The Centers for Disease Control (CDC) revised the guidelines for HIV screening and linkage, stating that patients should be screened at any point of entry into the healthcare system at least one time in their adult life. This number increased to once every six months if the patient had known high-risk features such as sex work, IV drug use, or men who have sex with men (Branson et al. 2006). The CDC policy disruption, while not an earthquake, did have aftershocks that included eventual changes in state legal requirements around HIV screening.

Until 2015, patients were required to tell physicians that they wanted HIV screening, referred to as "opt-in" testing. In 2015, Florida law shifted to allow for "opt-out" HIV testing, meaning that HIV screening became a part of routine ED care, though the patient had the right to tell the physician they did not want to be screened. This switch in screening model, along with relaxed guidelines around pre- and-posttest counseling created a new reality where HIV screening would be possible in the ED. Given this decreased barrier to HIV screening, as well as clarity around treatment initiation, an EM physician (JWW) felt a renewed urgency to scale up HIV screening in the Tampa General Hospital ED. Soon after the laws around opt-in testing were changed, this physician-anthropologist was able to build HIV screening into routine ED care through a partnership with the county Department of Health.

As this model was uncharted territory, the initial plan utilized third-party affiliates for HIV screening; those staff would come into the ED and offer rapid oral screening using saliva. The affiliates, unfortunately, were not able to identify many patients willing to be screened for HIV. The approach of a third-party worker with a seemingly, irrelevant, oral test seemed out of place with the current ED visit and standard workflow in acute care medicine (which utilizes serum-based testing for most disease states). For the first year (2015), approximately 65 oral HIV screening tests were conducted, identifying 2 HIV positive patients. Though a small percentage of patients were reached, this initial effort represented the first attempt at non-targeted ED-based screening (e.g., all patients that met CDC screening criteria) in the Tampa Bay area.

In 2016, an exponential shift occurred in ED-based HIV screening, when JWW was awarded funding to hire linkage to care and data coordination staff for the screening of both HIV and hepatitis C virus (HCV). In addition, this new source of funding paid for serum-based screening that could be more easily worked into the standard processes of ED care (e.g., blood draws for common laboratory analysis). This funding also allowed for the integration of HIV screening into the electronic medical record and a clinical decision support tool to facilitate physician computer order entry, greatly facilitating the opt-out testing process. Further, the hospital supported this screening by placing signage in every ED room that provided information on the screening process, notifying patients that they were able to opt out of HIV testing.

After conducting *zero* non-targeted HIV screening tests in 2014 (the year before ED-based screening was launched), and 65 in 2015, implementation of this new methodology and financial support resulted in 15,004 HIV tests in 2016, identifying 198 patients with HIV (including 7 that were newly positive and came to the ED with HIV infection-related symptoms). Since 2016, an additional 91,018 ED patients have been screened for HIV, identifying 764 patients with HIV. Of the 764 positives, 28 patients exhibited new viral symptoms, indicating an acute presentation of disease. Due to federal funding for HIV treatment that establishes clear linkage pathways for newly diagnosed patients, over 95% of these patients identified with HIV from the ED have been linked to care. Much of our early work screening and linking patients with HIV was done with the help of public health specialists under the guidance of a physician-anthropologist, but the specific contributions of anthropologists to design that care pathway were not definite. In other words, we had not yet maximized the value of a different perspective that medical anthropologists could bring to care pathway development and the work, while important, was based on established public health models.

The initial funding award for HIV screening and linkage also included screening and linkage for HCV. Traditionally, HCV was thought of as a virus with a declining prevalence, concentrated among "baby boomers" born between 1945 and 1965 ("age cohort"). The treatment for HCV, prior to 2015, was difficult to access and rarely successful (interferon [IFN]-based treatment had failure rates up to 50%). Since some patients with HCV cleared their own virus (around 20% per year), unlike HIV, coupled with the assumed prevalence decline due to an aging population, even less attention was paid to HCV screening and linkage by acute care and EM providers. However, the opioid epidemic shifted this epidemiology beginning in 2010 (CDC 2021) and, suddenly, our own screening data began to move toward a bimodal distribution of patients born in the age cohort (1945–1965) and patients born after 1980.

THE OPIOID EPIDEMIC IN THE UNITED STATES

Beginning in 2009, opioid-related ED encounters began to drastically increase (CDC 2020)—first driven by the pharmaceutical supply of drug and then the illicit heroin market after pill prescriptions became more tightly regulated. Finally, current increases in opioid-related encounters represent a mix of newer synthetic opioids, such as fentanyl, as well as heroin, hydromorphone (Dilaudid), and oxycodone. For over a decade, ED encounters related to OUD increased but EM physicians often discharged patients with, at best, phone numbers and addresses for abstinence-only costly inpatient rehabilitation facilities or methadone clinics (which were highly stigmatized patients presented, not well connected to acute care spaces and hard to gain access directly from an ED or hospital). ED-based treatment of opioid use disorder requires first rendering visible opioid use disorder patients as patients that belong in the ED. Medicalization of the opioid use itself allows consideration of treatment options (e.g., buprenorphine or methadone) and linkage to future care necessitates establishing providers and spaces for continued medically managed care that patients will trust.

STIGMA AND LEARNED HELPLESSNESS OF OPIOID USE DISORDER

Heather Henderson began work as a graduate student in the ED in 2016 and spent hundreds of hours conducting participant observation with patients that had opioid use disorder, as well as the physicians and healthcare teams that cared for those patients. Henderson recognized that healthcare team stigma related to opioid use disorder would have to be reduced to move to a medical model of disease management (Figure 10.1, Henderson 2018). Henderson's MA thesis work was key to our eventual development of a patient and provider informed care pathway model for the ED-based management of opioid use disorder. Key to Henderson's work, however, was also the emphasis on the social aspects of opioid dependence and withdrawal even in the frame of a medical model. Through patient interviews, Henderson uncovered a striking lack of healthcare access, prior criminality of dependence, and fear

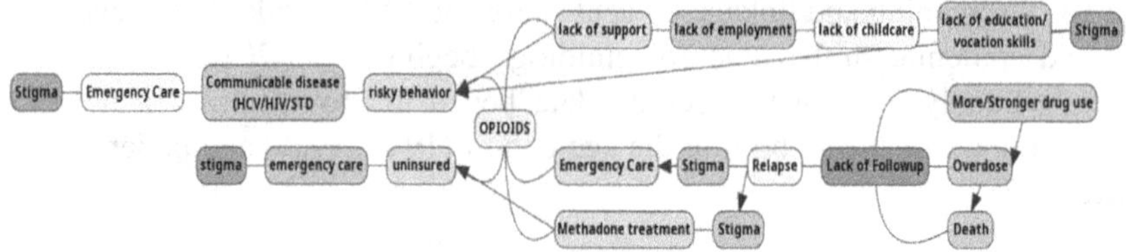

Figure 10.1 Stigma and the Dynamics of Opioid Use Disorder. *Source*: Reproduced from Henderson, H (2018). MA Thesis. University of South Florida.

of the healthcare system secondary to prior encounters. The prior management of opioid dependence was binary—if patients presented unconscious during an acute overdose, they might receive high doses of intravenous Narcan (an important reversal agent for opioids that would lead to recovery from respiratory depression but also painful precipitated withdrawal). The iatrogenic effects of the precipitated then led to many of these patients leaving the hospital against medical advice, requiring chemical restraints with IV antipsychotic medications to protect from self-harm (or even physical restrain) and then subsequent hospital admission secondary to restraint. At most, overdose patients were monitored for medical complications, sometimes necessitating admission to the ICU. If no overdose was present, many of these patients were simply discharged from the ED with a superficial list of resources after an "emergent medical condition" was not identified (even though one-year mortality after opioid overdose presentation to the ED may be as high as 5%).

"Stigma transforms addiction from a relapsing brain disease into a moral failing—laying the blame squarely on the person suffering addiction" (Henderson 2018:15). A medical model of addiction must remain informed by these social and structural realities to achieve success. Before Heather's work, there was very limited participant observation done by medical anthropologists and anthropology students at the acute crisis point of opioid withdrawal or during an acute care encounter. However, it is during these acute encounters where pathways might be most successful (patient has access to this space, patient may be engaged in healthcare decisions at that time) but are most lacking (limited access to these direct spaces and limited researchers engaging directly in applied clinical questions). While Henderson's work expectedly recounted the structural violence and traumatic life courses of patients with stigmatized disease, she also uncovered a learned helplessness that has been the key to further pathway development. Specifically, physicians, law enforcement, social workers, and patients, after years of lack of options and access, had largely given up on medical management of opioid dependence. Even though patients that present to the ED after an overdose have a mortality rate within the range of patients who present to the ED with a myocardial infarct, around 5% at one year (Larochelle et al. 2018; Weiner et al. 2020), very little was done for these patients prior to new modes of pathway development. As we grappled with the syndemic links between opioid dependence and HCV (Singer 2009), Henderson's ethnographic insights have served as the foundation for our interventions (Henderson 2018).

HCV AND YOUNG PEOPLE WHO INJECT DRUGS

The epidemiological shift to a bimodal distribution (e.g., HCV infection in "baby boomer" age cohort and among people born after 1980) has tracked areas with higher opioid use. Restrictions on opioid prescribing and the availability of large quantities of opioids through pill mills accelerated the epidemic by driving patients to heroin and other non-pharmaceutically available opioid options (CDC 2021). People Who Inject Drugs (PWID) now make up over 90% of new cases of HCV and pose new challenges for screening and linkage to treatment (CDC 2021). While our screening program continues to observe a high prevalence of HCV among those born after 1980, with over 4,296 cases of HCV identified since 2015 from 2016 to 2018, only 50% of patients were successfully linked to treatment; much less than the 95% rate observed for patients with HIV.

HISTORY OF HCV TREATMENT

Before 2015, IFN was the only medical treatment available for HCV but led to poor outcomes (low efficacy for viral response in patients that completed course of IFN with side effects commonly reported). Furthermore, HCV testing requires a two-step process of first identifying a positive antibody and then confirming the presence of active virus by an RNA PCR test. HCV treatment and testing have never been part of ED-based, or even acute hospital, patient management. However, those with opioid use disorder, epidemiologically, have an HCV problem—either the patient has HCV or will have HCV with continued IV drug use. In addition, those with detectable HCV RNA can easily transmit HCV to other members of needle sharing networks as HCV "lives" easily on drug paraphernalia.

Direct acting antivirals (DAAs) now offer accessible treatment options that lead to sustained viral response (SVR) within two to three months in patients with chronic HCV (Feld 2015). Even though this treatment is available, providers have been skeptical regarding utilizing the medication in patients with ongoing or recent opioid use disorder. Available data though suggest efficacy without the development of resistance or recurrence of HCV after the use of DAAs in PWID (Cunningham et al. 2018).

PWID AND HCV TREATMENT

In 2018, patients enrolled in the SIMPLIFY trial (Grebeley et al. 2018) demonstrated that PWID that completed 12 weeks of DAA treatment achieved the same rates of SVR (> 95%) as birth cohort and non-PWID patients, pragmatically confirming guidelines which suggest the use of DAAs in PWID. Even though guidelines suggest DAAs should be used in PWID patients with HCV (Ghany et al. 2020), low DAA use in PWID may be secondary to perceived fears of reinfection and drug resistance, cost, unknown future of patient's HCV (some patients will clear the disease themselves), difficulty of ensuring follow-up in vulnerable people, and, potentially, lack of deservingness and considered moral failures of HCV patients who inject drugs.

ENTANGLEMENT: HCV, OPIOIDS, AND CAPITALIST RUINS ENCOUNTER THE ED

Opioid use disorder is entangled in whiteness, education, labor, capitalism, hospitals, suffering, belonging, physicians, but also ensnares infectious disease acutely and chronically (e.g., hepatitis and HIV). Altogether, this entanglement of (non)medicalized models, viruses, drugs, drug manufacturers, patients, physicians, treatments, paraphernalia represent an assemblage. Modern approaches in ED-based care disentangle the opioid use disorder and reject the notion of belonging in patients who are "not sick" or focus on the phenotypic expression of overdose, treating the hemodynamics but not the underlying dependence or addiction. Ironically, by working to medicalize these assemblages, what is thought of as an illness may appear instead as a fundamentally disproportionate distribution of resources (Lynn-Callo 2000). In other words, by elevating opioid use disorder to a medicalized condition, the patients are not only visualized, but the causes of the opioid use, the overdose, and the lack of treatment begin to appear rooted in cultural, structural, and social determinants, inviting those domains into the clinical space as well.

Our initial linkage to care rates following positive screening for HCV in the ED were only 25% (compared to our HIV linkage rates of 90%). Low rates of linkage were largely due to the difficulty of resulting patients (e.g., contacting patients to inform them of the positive result and to discuss follow-up options), difficulty establishing a follow-up location (e.g., lack of primary care, lack of health insurance), and difficulty in patients showing up for scheduled visits. HCV screening and linkage interviews also, incidentally, served as screening for injection drug use and illustrated an increasing frequency of PWID in the ED.

In 2017, we recognized a need to establish a pathway for PWID given the high volume of PWID diagnoses in the ED and the concern for HCV transmission between needle sharing networks of patients given the high seroprevalence of virus in the population (about 70% in our cohort). Following the work of D'Onofrio et al. (2015), JWW and HH established the region's first ED-based medically assisted therapy program (now known as medication for opioid use disorder, MOUD) and began initiating buprenorphine in the ED and linking patients to a trusted community substance use facility for continued care in September 2018.

MEDICAL MANAGEMENT FOR OPIOID USE DISORDER

Methadone, a medication for management of opioid use disorder, usually requires on-site dispensing at an approved methadone clinic. Thus, methadone has not been considered an option for initiation of therapy, maintenance of withdrawal, or for opioid use disorder patients that present to the ED. Buprenorphine (Suboxone, Subutex) was FDA approved for use in the United States in 1981. However, according to the Narcotic Addiction Treatment Act of 1974 (S. 115, Govtrack.us), any physician that treats opiate addiction must obtain a separate registration. For buprenorphine, this registration is in the form of the "X-Waiver" (DATA 2000) which is still required at the time of this writing (Bliley HR 2634, 2000).

An ED-based landmark trial by EM physicians D'Onofrio and colleagues, published in 2015, demonstrated that when patients received buprenorphine in the ED, rates of treatment engagement 10 weeks later were higher than in groups that received only the standard of care (screening and referral) as well as patients that received both screening and referral as well as a brief, focused intervention. The trial has generated new research approaches to ED-based buprenorphine pathways and increased DATA 2000 waiver accessibility and training (BUPE 2021) for emergency physicians.

More recently, acute care physicians (e.g., EM, intensivists, internists) have utilized the "three-day rule" in Title 21, CFR 1306.07(b) ("Three Day Rule," DEA) to initiate buprenorphine treatment in the ED and hospital to stabilize patients in acute opioid withdrawal. Withdrawal can be measured using a validated clinical opioid withdrawal score (COWS) (Wesson et al. 2003; Tompkins et al. 2009). A patient is in active withdrawal if COWS is greater than four (MDCalc.com 2021) and those patients may benefit from acute use of buprenorphine in the ED. Word of mouth and anecdotal success with this strategy to stabilize ED patients with opioid withdrawal began to spread across the EM community in the early 2010s (personal observation) and formal research studies into ED-based buprenorphine pathways were initiated as the medical model of drug dependence as a chronic, relapsing, disease state also spread throughout the discipline (McLellan et al. 2000).

ED-BASED MOUD AND HCV TREATMENT PATHWAY

In September 2018, HH and JWW initiated an ED-based MOUD pathway, stabilizing patients in the ED with COWS > = 4 with a one-time dose of buprenorphine and then linkage to care same day or next at an established community partner facility to continue MOUD. As of March 2021, after 30 months of program operation, over 600 patients have been able to access MOUD and have been successfully linked to treatment in the community. The success rate for linking OUD patients to care remains around 70%, 48% higher than the national average of 22% for the establishment of care after an ED visit (Mancher and Leshner 2019). The success of this treatment pathway has vastly improved clinical care for this patient population, and was made possible by utilizing an anthropological frame, paired with the integration of patients' lived experiences of what historically happened when trying to access care; these lived experiences were built directly into pathway design (HH). Today, the number of MOUD pathway patients that are HCV positive remains around 70%. By building a clear path to treatment for those suffering from opioid use disorder, patients will now also have access to HCV medical treatment as well.

THE ANTHROPOLOGICAL DIFFERENCE: EXTENDING SYNDEMICS AND COLOCATING TREATMENT

Working with a Federally Qualified Healthcare Center that is located on-site at the substance disorder treatment facility, we established a pilot program in which patients with HCV and MOUD are offered DAA therapy for HCV. Ideally, early treatment of HCV among PWID decreased HCV transmission and downstream rates of cirrhosis and hepatocellular carcinoma. This program, as far as we know, is the one the first time HCV + PWID patients have initiated MOUD concomitantly with DAAs for HCV in a formal pathway. The concomitant treatment strategy is an extended syndemic model, moving from description to treatment (Singer et al. 2017).

We have already outlined the entangled nature of opioid dependence with biomedicine, neoliberal capitalism, poverty, structural violence, stigma, and learned helplessness. The drivers of opioid dependence become the drivers of HCV infection as new infections occur primarily in PWID. Singer et al. (2009, 2017) have previously outlined the concept of syndemics that has been summarized and adopted by the CDC (2001) as

> health related problems [that] cluster by person, place or time. The problems—along with the reasons for their clustering—define a syndemic and differentiate one from another. To prevent a syndemic, one must not only prevent or control each disease but also the forces that tie those diseases together. (CDC 2001, Henderson 2018)

Our work moves syndemic descriptions of disease to syndemically informed construction of new assemblages for patient care and treatment (Singer et al. 2017).

Recognition of assemblage formations (point of time and space occurrence in ED of structural, pathophysiologic, current political context, trends in biomedicine, specific treating physician, overall care team, preestablished pathway, patient lived experiences, embodiment and expression of illness), scenes and patches of patient disease, also invites the creation of new pathways for patient care (a previously unconsidered pathway to initiate medications for opioid use disorder in the ED, concomitant treatment of opioid use disorder and hepatitis C infection, new drug delivery for sickle cell disease pain crisis). At times, those pathways must consider structural and social forces that synergize disease risk and expression (e.g., syndemics). Novel new strategies may consider treatment of disease along these pathways, addressing structural vulnerability, ensuring systemic and provider structural competencies, and even colocating care when syndemic assemblages are identified (e.g., HCV and opioid use disorder treatment at same time and place). Syndemic approaches do not need to be invoked for every assemblage but do provide a way to conceptualize new assemblage formations and methods for disentanglement. Furthermore, not all assemblages of suffering can be medicalized, even when encountering the healthcare system. Trying to do this runs into the challenge faced by homeless shelter staff in Lyon-Callo's work: "We can't change the economy, so we have to change you" (Lyon-Callo 2000).

Physician participation in patient-centered care pathways may resolve the tension between a failed modern biomedical system and the other ways that patients continue to demand and seek relief of suffering. Syndemic models can not only describe disease processes (IVDU, HCV) and relationships with social forces (post-capitalist despair, whiteness, education) but, moving into a new space, also inform treatment strategies unimagined previously (e.g., co-treatment of opioid use disorder and HCV in same space and time).

CONCLUSIONS

If physicians are to engage in new ontologies of suffering and care (expressed through active participation in creating new pathways and models of disease identification and treatment), biomedical education must embrace structural competencies early in medical education and drive patient-centered approaches to suffering (e.g., patient shadowing, curriculum emphasizing structural competency, medical anthropologist role modeling in clinical settings). If biomedical healthcare is to play a role in relief of suffering, the tension between the failed models of healthcare must be resolved.

Our HIV and HCV linkage program has expanded to include treatment of opioid use disorder and HCV. This expansion has developed our approach to care pathways as a way to solve "learned helplessness" of patients and physicians that exist within healthcare systems that have largely reified specific health inequities. Our approach to pathway development draws on anthropological concepts that date back to Kleinman's explanatory models of disease and illness but are also informed by newer understandings of entanglements and assembles. Specifically, we are evaluating our extension of syndemic models as descriptives of disease to potential ways to approach colocated disease management.

Our work continues to expand pathways focused on decreasing deaths from opioid use and the transmission of HCV. We initiated a free naloxone (Narcan) program in 2019 that distributes the reversal agent for opioids in the ED and among our nascent needle exchange program. Each time we hand out Narcan, we provide a self-addressed stamped envelope and ask those that use the lifesaving drug to return the postcard to us anonymous to record use. In a one-year period of time, we distributed 600 kits and documented 284 overdose reversals. Figure 10.2 demonstrates the impact of this program—an impact we have shared with healthcare providers and other funding stakeholders as recognition of the positive and promising work they are doing.

We launched (JWW and HH) the second legal sterile syringe program (SSP in the state following the Florida Infectious Disease Elimination Act) (Florida DOH 2017). IDEA Tampa was approved in February 2020 (Cordoba-Perez 2020) in Hillsborough County, Florida, and went live in January 2021. Florida law, prior to 2017, did not allow for needle exchange harm reduction programs. However, a pilot program needle exchange was allowed in Miami-Dade County. The exchange quickly demonstrated identification of an HIV outbreak and based on those successes, the state legislature later cleared

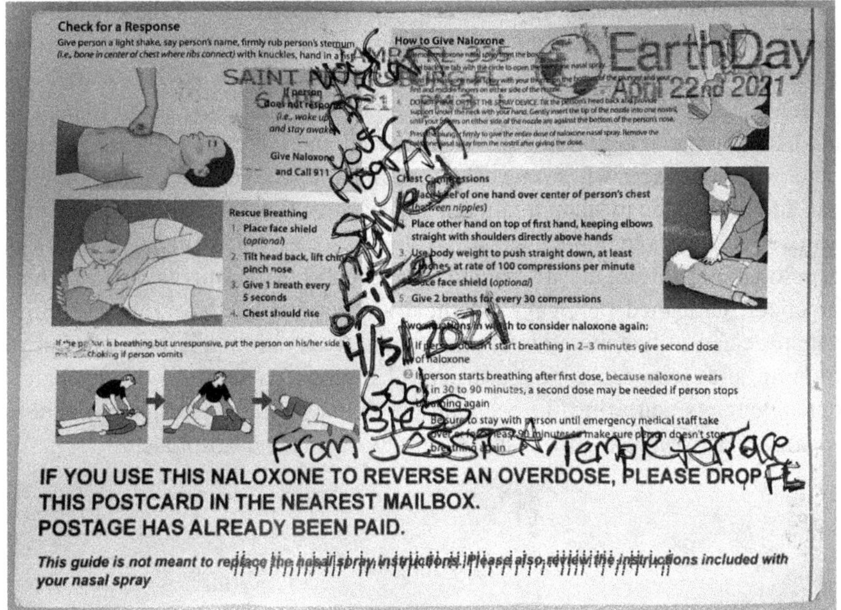

Figure 10.2 Naloxone Reversal and Instruction Postcard Returned to Our Group after Use. *Source*: Postcard Created by Heather Henderson and Jason Wilson.

the way for counties to approve one-to-one sterile syringe program in each county (Tookes et al. 2019).

Our syringe services program, in collaboration with Dr. Asa Oxner of University of South Florida Tampa Bay Street Medicine, operates five days per week with needle exchange services, partnerships with other key groups (e.g., sex worker representatives), anonymous and confidential HIV testing and HCV testing. We are entering our sixth year of HIV/HCV ED-based screening and linkage, have expanded the program to a satellite ED, and work closely with the county as members of the Health Care Advisory Board (JWW), the Opioid Task Force (JWW and HH), and the Behavioral Task Force to advise, consult, and recommend best practices for eliminating infectious disease, working with patients that have opioid use disorder and designing enhanced harm reduction strategies that remove stigma long held against these patient populations. We are now fully integrated into the hospital and function as a division within the ED; JWW serves as one of the department medical directors, and HH, a medical anthropologist, serves as the director of Social Medicine, a division within the ED created in 2019. In 2020 that division expanded with the hiring of our first postdoctoral applied medical anthropologist (BLM) as associate division director.

We continue to expand the idealized space and structure of the ED, as well as the type of patient that belongs and deserves care by hardwiring existing patient pathways we created and establishing more new ways to see and treat patients. We believe that our general approach to pathway development in the ED can extend beyond opioid use disorder and infectious disease and into other medical spaces where critical, clinically applied medical anthropologists can add high value to static treatment approaches. Sickle cell disease and firearm violence are other areas we are exploring for new and enhanced pathway development. Physicians are trained to select and treat patients based on best practice established pathways. Medical anthropologists working in a clinical space can utilize methods of participant observation and their theoretical training and perspective (e.g., structural violence, structural determinants, entanglements, suffering) to cocreate previously unimagined patient-centric treatment pathways in partnership with physicians and hospitals.

Chapter 11

Firearm Research

In this chapter we report on preliminary results of a research study on patients who present to the Emergency Department (ED) with nonfatal gunshot wounds (NFGSWs). In doing so, we begin to move between clinical and public health/policy spaces. We broaden our concept of cultural differences between physician/provider and patient (Kleinman et al. 1978) to that of public health versus community perspective. We feel that further understanding of how and why people are shot is critical to the development of effective programs and policies to prevent such injuries. This follows a long tradition in medical anthropology which calls for understanding the community perspective on the nature of the problem before designing an effective public health program/policy (Yasumaro et al. 1998). This topic is also a useful one in which to consider the roles of both cultural and structural issues related to these injuries.

BACKGROUND

Gun violence in the United States has been considered a national public health concern since the early 1990s (Koop and Lundberg 1992). More recently, this public health issue has reached a considerable amount of public attention in the context of mass shooting events across the country, even though mass shootings represent only a small proportion of overall firearm fatalities (Fox and Fridel 2016). To date, gun violence research has predominantly employed epidemiological approaches with quantitative analyses (Wintemute 2015; Sherman 2001) with a paucity of qualitative studies that use ethnographic methods and that are specifically conducted in a medical setting, although work by Metzl (2018); Richardson, Vil, and

Cooper (2015, 2016); Rich (2009) and Ralph (2014) has made important contributions in that space.

The existing body of literature regarding gun violence has predominantly focused on the epidemiological nature of these traumatic events (Fox and Fridel 2018; Wintemute 2015; Sherman 2001; Koop and Lundberg 1992). These studies have additionally focused on broad policy-based interventions in addressing the issue (Wintemute 2015). While these types of interventions have generally contributed to the relative decrease in the prevalence of traumatic events and deaths as a result of gun violence since the 1980s and 1990s, the past decade has seen a rapidly growing number of these same types of events (Wintemute 2015). This public health issue becomes more difficult in addressing universally, when considering the contextual differences across different states, counties, and individual communities (different laws regarding firearm access). This is where applied social scientific approaches to studying gun violence become more critical in ethnographically understanding the rise in gun violence incidents across the country and, potentially, how to craft informed intervention strategies.

Even though the United States contains less than 5% of the world population, the country is home to over 40% of the firearms in the world. Over the past three decades, there has been a disproportionately small amount of firearm-related research given the clinical burden and economic impact of gunshot wound injuries when compared to other disease states and public health issues facing Americans like cancer, HIV, motor vehicle crashes, sepsis, myocardial infarcts, and strokes. Firearm safety and firearm violence data has been difficult to obtain secondary to nonuniform crime reporting statistics and actual restrictions on funding for firearm research. Kellerman et al. (1993) linked the presence of guns in homes to an increased risk of homicide. That study was a compelling quantitative analysis demonstrating that guns represented a public health risk and suggested further hypothesis testing would be needed. The results of that study have held up. In a 2007 analysis, the higher the percent of households with firearms in a state, the higher the incidence of firearm-related mortality in that state (Miller et al. 2007). In addition, a 2013 study demonstrated that for every percentage point increase in gun ownership, there was a concomitant 0.9% increase in the firearm homicide rate (Siegel et al. 2013). However, The National Rifle Association (NRA) has lobbied to inhibit the ability of researchers to conduct scientific studies on guns, gun safety, and gun violence by inserting language into the 1996 omnibus spending bill. The rider was authored by Republican Congressman Jay Dickey and referred to as the Dickey Amendment. The Dickey Amendment specifically restricted injury prevention research funding leading to "gun control" (itself a pejorative and poorly defined term). This restriction was in affect from 1996 until 2020 when 26 million dollars was finally allocated into the federal budget and directed toward firearm research. The Dickey Amendment had a crushing impact on firearm safety research, decreasing federal funding by 96% as well as peer-reviewed publications by 60% over the next 20 years (Metzl 2018).

The 26-million-dollar allocation in 2020 occurred only after a number of pivotal events unfolded during the past decade including multiple high-profile mass shootings involving children (Sandy Hook, Parkland), unsuspecting adults at entertainment venues (Las Vegas) as well as at numerous workplaces and shopping centers. Even though mass shootings (five or more people killed during a single encounter) account for only a small proportion of the total number of individuals killed each year by firearms, the headlines and terror that result have had a lasting public impression.

The Dickey Amendment not only prohibited firearm safety research but also damaged the attempts by firearm safety advocates for a public health model of gun safety and attempts to equate regulations and laws that decrease firearm death and injury to similar laws that were designed after the advent of automobiles aimed at decreasing high levels of morbidity and mortality from car crashes. In 1946, there were 9.35 fatalities for every 100 million vehicle miles traveled. Cars were not banned but instead seatbelts, safety standards, speed limits, child seats, airbags, and mandatory defect laws were all developed, decreasing car crash–related fatalities to 1.18 per 100 million vehicle miles traveled (NHTSA 2010). Cars are a would-be analogy to how the United States might have approached gun safety and firearm violence. However, the NRA is a powerful lobby and has pushed lawmakers to avoid regulations in the face of overwhelming public support for specific gun safety–related regulations.

Just as the public assassination attempt of Ronald Regan in the 1980s led to the widespread support of the Brady Bill after Regan's aid, James Brady was permanently disabled by a gunshot wound; the public also overwhelmingly supports universal background checks following a string of mass shooting events during the 2010s. Polls have consistently estimated 80% to 89% support for "red flag" laws that would restrict some gun purchases in cases of prior interpersonal violence convictions, prior gun crime convictions, or mental health flags (APM 2019). Red flag laws (universal background checks, removing guns from individuals deemed to be dangerous by a court, restrictions on high-capacity ammunition clips, and even bans on semiautomatic weapons, and the technology to easily create automatic weapons such as bump stocks) all have majority support in the United States. Twenty-two percent of firearms are purchased without a background check (Miller et al. 2017). Bump stocks serve little purpose outside of rapid human killing and were used in the Las Vegas nightclub shootings. A bump stock allows a trigger to be held down, essentially converting a semiautomatic weapon to an automatic weapon (figure 11.1). Other public health style regulations that have polled well among the public include raising the age of firearm purchases to 21, safe storage requirements (e.g., mandatory trigger locks), smart guns (if my iPhone only works for me, why doesn't my gun behave in the same way?), allow lawsuits against firearm companies, limitations on the number of guns that can be bought each month by one individual as well as ammunition checks that limit the amount of ammunition purchased as well as background checks on those purchasing ammunition (APM 2019).

Regardless of straw man arguments to the contrary from gun rights lobbyist groups, there is still a correlation between guns in households and increased incidents of homicide, often secondary to interpersonal violence. In addition, putting the common "a lot of gun homicides occur in Chicago" (Chicago Tribune 2017) arguments to the side (because Chicago is a city close to multiple states with lax gun laws and also a city in the United States that exists within a context of other structural problems that lead to intercity violence, as well as state-sanctioned asymmetrical violence by law enforcement), there is data that clearly demonstrates that fewer guns lead to fewer deaths and tighter gun restrictions lead to both fewer guns and fewer deaths.

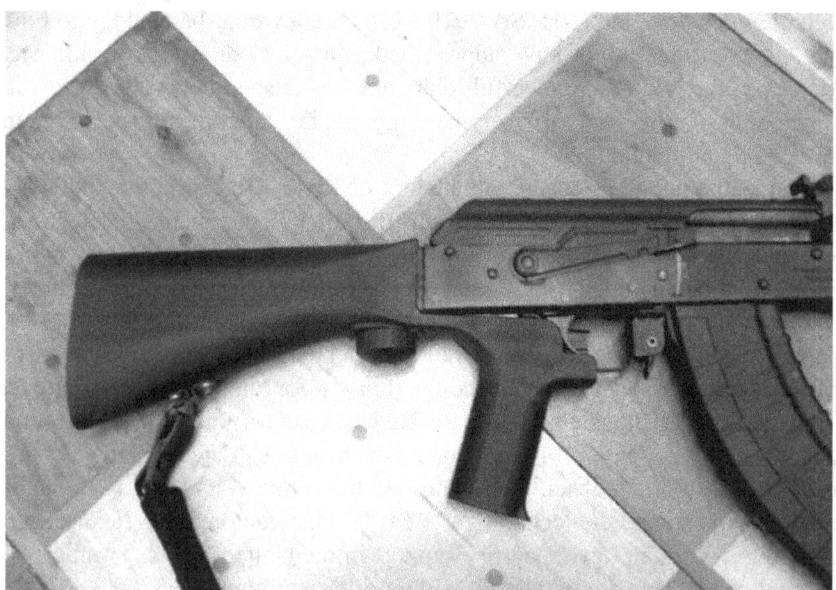

Figure 11.1 The Bump Stock Allows the Trigger to Stay Depressed Essentially Converting a Semiautomatic Weapon to an Automatic Weapon. *Source*: Created by WASR. Wikipedia. ShareAlike 3.0 Unported (CC BY-SA 3.0). No changes made.

Unfortunately, given the limitations of gun safety research and gun safety data, suicides by firearm often must be used as a proxy for gun ownership (Rabin 2020). In addition, even when considering Chicago as a part of Illinois, the state has a below average amount of gun-related deaths (9/100K), in line with other states that have implemented a higher-than-average amount of gun regulations (Chicago Tribune 2017). Put another way, the Law Center to Prevent Gun Violence/Gifford Law Center rates Illinois a "A-," along with Rhode Island, Washington, and Delaware. B states have average gun deaths of 8.13/100k (compared to A states with 5.22/100K and the United States average of 10.5/100K) (Gifford Law Center 2021).

A common refrain to the public health approach to gun safety is that one specific public health initiative would not have prevented another specific shooting or event. Public health operates in a combination of strategies which, together, bring down rates of undesired events—sexually transmitted infections, maternal death, rates of premature birth, car crash fatalities, chronic disease–related deaths, and so on. All of the public health interventions focused on improving gun safety will not completely erase all gun deaths, but, together, they will drastically decrease firearm fatality rates. Of note, another gun rights lobby argument is that if people want to kill others or kill themselves, they will find a way to do so; however, there is no data to support this assertion and a preponderance of evidence suggesting the opposite is true (there are less homicides and fewer suicides when there are fewer guns).

FIREARM–RELATED SUICIDE

Of course, another reason why arguments about "Chicago" or suggestions that people always find ways to kill others, or that some mass shootings would have still occurred even with tighter gun safety laws, are beside the point is that the highest fatal use of firearms is from suicide. Firearm-related suicides are completed at a much higher rate than non-firearm related suicides as they allow for impulse decisions, often while individuals are intoxicated. Delaying access (e.g., gun locks) and reducing the number of guns in homes would decrease the approximately 22,000 suicides by gun that occur each year (about two-thirds of gun-related deaths). Even though firearms are only used in 6% of suicide attempts, guns are responsible for 50% of all suicide deaths (Miller et al. 2008). In addition, firearm-related suicides occur at a rate 10 times higher compared to other high-income countries (Grinshteyn et al. 2019). While the gun lobby has suggested that a high incidence of gun-related deaths take place through black-on-black homicide, the reality is that homicides account for only one-third of gun-related deaths, and among those homicides approximately 43% take place among family members or other

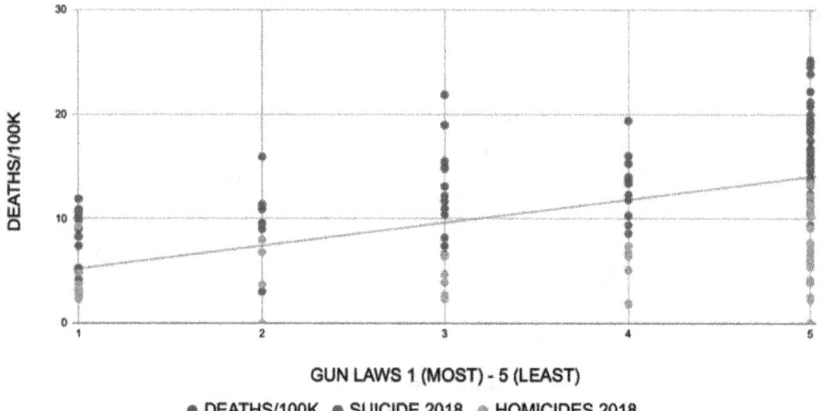

Figure 11.2 Created Using Publicly Available CDC Data for Homicide and Suicide Deaths by Gun. *Source*: Figure created by Jason Wilson. Data from CDC WONDER Database (CDC 2019).

relationships (FBI Data), meaning only 22% of gun fatalities are related to unknown assailant firearm injuries, fitting the category of peer "black-on-black crime" popularized in gun advocacy talking points. More important, 72% of all homicides involve a firearm (FBI data) and fewer guns are associated with fewer homicides. As with suicide, homicides are more difficult to complete and less likely without a gun and are less common in states with increased firearm safety regulations. Figure 11.2 illustrates a relationship between states with tighter gun purchasing and gun safety laws and the incidence of suicide and homicide-related firearm mortality. While another faulty argument is that gun laws will only stop "good guys" from getting guns, the lower number of gun-related deaths in states with increased gun laws demonstrates that fewer guns in circulation also leads to fewer "bad guys" with guns when considering the homicide-related fatalities. Of course, suicides drive two-thirds of the gun-related fatalities so this is essentially a moot argument anyway if the discussion is focused on a public health approach to decreasing all-cause gun-related deaths.

Suicide completion takes place at the highest rates among white males with a firearm (Harvard 2016). White males make up 86% of firearm-related suicide deaths and white male suicides with a gun make up 58% of all suicides. Metzl has outlined the relationship between whiteness (and maleness) in his book *Dying of Whiteness* (2019a) which outlines how racism drives white Americans to vote against their own interests, literally increasing death rates from gun violence (suicide), drug use, and addiction as well as decreased financial mobility through failing schools and less education opportunities. Metzl considers his home state of Missouri as an example of how gun safety regulations were decreased over time resulting in an overall increase in suicide deaths by white men, centering the increase in suicides as a public health and political problem, not solely a mental health crisis. From 2012 to 2019, the suicide rate increased in Missouri by 25% from 14.3/100K to 18.9/100K (Metzl 2019a).

Overall, suicides have exponentially increased in the United States beginning in 2001 (Curtain et al., 2016). This increase was driven by white men (figure 11.3). This increase in deaths among whites, especially whites without a college education, has been quantitatively documented by Case and Deaton (2015, 2020) who demonstrated that life expectancy has declined in non-Hispanic whites without a college education. More specifically, deaths during middle age among non-Hispanic whites without at least a bachelor's degree have driven down overall life expectancy in the United States. Beginning at the turn of the twenty-first century, life expectancy stopped increasing (or mortality rates stopped falling) in the United States compared to other high-income countries. Breaking this down further, mortality among college-educated whites changed very little while mortality among blacks continued to decline as racist policies and structural barriers to health continued to fall throughout the end of the twentieth and beginning of the twenty-first

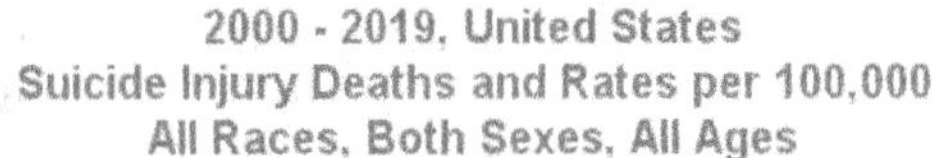

2000 - 2019, United States
Suicide Injury Deaths and Rates per 100,000
All Races, Both Sexes, All Ages

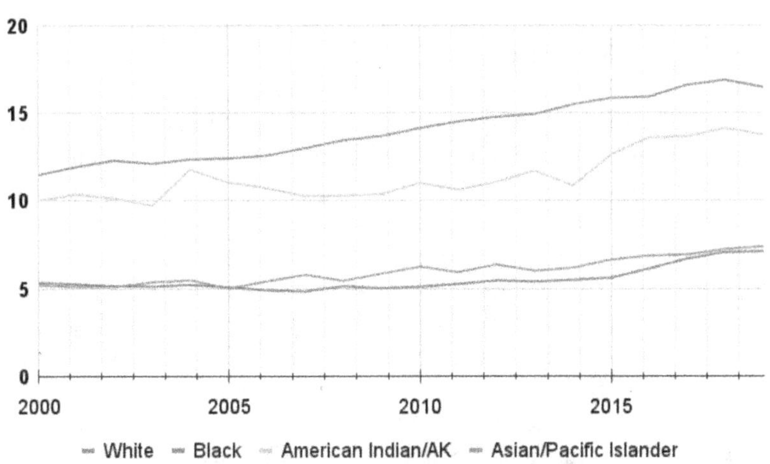

Figure 11.3 Suicide Rates by Race in the United States. *Source*: Figure created by Jason Wilson. Data source: WISQARS Fatal Injury Reports, National, Regional, and State, 1981–2019, CDC.

century, increasing the life expectancy for people of color. The increased mortality among non-Hispanic Whites without a college degree in middle age (age-adjusted mortality) began in the late 1990s and is not simply explained away by the terrorist attack of 9/11 or the 2008 recession. Instead, Case and Deaton show quantitatively that increases in suicides and drug addiction have occurred since the late 1990s (2015, 2020). While Case and Deaton describe the "what" (increasing rates of suicides among middle-age non-Hispanic Whites), Metzl's (2019b) policy analysis and interviews describe the "why" (decreasing gun safety regulations, protection of whiteness, and a history of racism in public policy, law, and medicine). Tying this together is the history of racist gun policies that favored gun ownership among whites over blacks that is so strongly protected even today those whites now drive down overall life expectancy in the United States.

GUN DENSITY AND SAFETY

Comparative state data demonstrates that fewer guns, not more guns, make a state safer. Of course, there are no state checkpoints or physical interstate boundaries that keep firearms from moving from a Grade F gun safety regulation state to a Grade A gun safety regulation state (Gifford Law Center 2021). However, there are data available across countries demonstrating the impact of gun safety regulations on firearm mortality. Australia serves as an excellent case example as the country is an island continent with uniform laws across the entire region, making entry of firearms into the area difficult compared to the heterogeneous state laws found throughout the United States. In the past, Australia had fairly unrestrictive gun laws. However, the Port Arthur mass shooting even in 1996 (35 dead, 23 wounded) led to sweeping changes in gun safety laws including a ban on rapid fire weapons, gun buyback programs as well licensing requirements for gun purchases along with background checks. While mass shootings do not drive the majority of gun-related deaths, the number of mass shootings declined from 13 in the 20 years prior to gun law changes to none in the 20 years after those new laws were passed (Chapman 2016). From a public health standpoint, the incidence of all-cause homicides and suicides must also decrease in order to suggest that improved gun safety regulations had a beneficial impact on mortality. While the suicide rate by firearm was already falling in Australia prior to the 1996 legal changes, the largest declines were seen after new gun safety laws were passed as firearm-related suicides in Australia decreased from 2.25/100K in 1995 to 1.1/100K in 2012 (Harvard 2011). Of note, even the pre-1996 rate of suicides was four times less than the states with the lowest suicide rates in the United States in 2018 (New Jersey and New York each had 8.3/100K). Homicide rates in

Australia also fell and declined most in areas of Australia that saw the highest participation in gun buyback programs. In 1996, homicide rates were around 0.5/100K (already in the group of states in the United States with the lowest homicide rates: Rhode Island, Maine, and Vermont) and decreased to 0.1/100K following increased firearm regulations.

The best similar comparisons in the United States have come from comparisons between Missouri (decreased gun regulations led to increased suicides and homicides) and Connecticut (increased gun regulations led to decreased suicides and increased homicides) since these states are geographically far enough away to hinder interstate movement of firearms to get around state laws and also saw policy changes begin moving in the opposite direction long enough ago to have post-intervention data but not so long ago that socio-cultural factors would have been markedly different or that data collection processes were dissimilar (Metzl 2019a). In 1995, Connecticut tightened gun purchasing requirements leading to a decrease of homicides by 40% over the following 20 years as well as a 15% decline in suicides. Meanwhile, beginning in 2007, Missouri has relaxed gun purchasing regulations, and since that time there has been a 25% increase in homicide rates and a 16% increase in suicide rates (Metzl 2019a).

PUBLIC HEALTH APPROACH TO REDUCING FIREARM DEATHS

An attempt at a public health approach has been put forward by multiple medical and professional societies but was roundly rejected by the NRA. A policy statement crafted by a number of medical societies in November 2018 and supporting some of these red flag laws was also determined to be in alignment with the second amendment protection of the right to bear arms in the United States (Butkus et al. 2018). The policy document was endorsed by the American College of Physicians, along with the American Academy of Family Medicine, American Academy of Pediatrics, American College of Obstetrical Gynecology, and even the American Bar Association. However, following the publication of this position paper, the NRA fought back against the objective medical approach, firing off a tweet that told, "self-important anti-gun doctors to stay in their lane."

In the environment of social media, sometimes the most directed challenges backfire. In the 12 hours after posting, the hashtag #ThisIsOurLane went viral. This demonstrated the possibility of an apolitical approach to gun safety, as many physicians not normally engaged in social justice entered into the ongoing social media discussion, calling first for their right to be expert members of the conversation and, second, for increased gun safety regulation to end the effects of firearm violence seen on a daily basis by Emergency Medicine, trauma surgery, and critical care specialist physicians (Ranney et al. 2019). The tweet damaged the NRA's reputation among even gun-owning physicians and others who recognized the first-hand experiences physicians have with gun violence and the genuine desire to decrease harm related to firearm injuries. Momentum from the viral tweet war (#StayinYourLane, @NRA vs. #ThisIsOurLane, thousands of physicians) led to the development of a private, nonprofit, gun safety research organization, the American Foundation for Firearm Injury Reduction in Medicine under the leadership of emergency physician and chief research officer, Megan Ranney. Ranney often states that the organization is not anti-gun; they are anti-shooting (seemingly a message that is apolitical).

QUANTITATIVE AND POPULATION LEVEL FIREARM VIOLENCE AND INJURY DATA

The lack of a coherent strategy, driven by federal funding and federal guidelines, along with the lack of uniform data has left gun researchers largely trying to capture quantitative evidence of firearm-related data: a skill well suited to public health researchers. Thus, the scant research over the past three decades has mostly been at the population level using quantitative results. Megan Ranney and colleagues at the American College of Emergency Physicians did outline a consensus statement, paving the way for future firearm safety research goals in 2017 (Ranney et al. 2017).

NFGSW

Ranney et al. (2017) identified that over 630 million dollars a year were spent on healthcare and legal-related consequences of NFGSW survivors. In addition, many of these NFGSW survivors encounter physicians in the ED, potentially serving as a place and time for a harm reduction intervention strategy. Specifically, signals that NFGSW injuries may represent an important area of investigation secondary to the disproportionate representation of this outcome of non-suicide related firearm violence, the high financial and emotional costs over time, as well as the realization that victims of NFGSW are at increased risk of firearm mortality and future gun violence–related events have been identified as important areas of further analysis by Kalesan and colleagues as well (Kalesan 2017). In 2014, there were 114,633 firearm-related injuries. Of those, 70% resulted in NFGSW, again suggesting that a significant opportunity for reduction of future violence may be positioned in further analysis of NFGSW survivors who may inform intervention strategies and represent a significant public health disease burden (Ranney et al. 2017). Kalesan et al. (2017) have shown that, over a 13-year period from 2001 to 2013, NFGSW injuries occurred at a rate of 23.4/100K in the United States. During this 13-year period, the rate of fatal gunshot wounds did not increase significantly (stable at 10.5/100K) while the incidence of NFGSW injuries has gone up by 17% (22.1/100K to 26.7/100K).

Carter et al. (2015) demonstrated that young people who present to the ED with a NFGSW are at increased for future mortality, while work by Lyons et al. (2019) adds to the treatment of a NFGSW as a sentinel event, recognizing the increased risk of that person for future firearm violence (Lyons et al. 2019). Lyons et al. (2019) suggest that the ED encounter, or during the hospital admission, could be a time to utilize a motivational, behavioral modification intervention to reduce future risk. Motivational interviewing has been successfully used during acute encounters with success, including among patients presenting to the hospital for alcohol intoxication (Gentilello et al. 1999). NFGSW injuries are a visual, economic, emotional avenue for firearm safety work that can help guide future hypothesis testing and also potentially save the lives of people already injured through firearm violence. In addition, the ability to more easily conduct firearm research in limited funding settings may invite the opportunity to work with victims of NFGSW injuries through social sciences approaches that also bridge gaps in medicine and public health strategies.

SOCIAL SCIENCE AND FIREARM VIOLENCE RESEARCH

Over the past three decades, social science approaches to firearm violence have also been implemented as they cost less and often ask questions oriented toward framing the issues within a social and cultural context. In addition, mixed method approaches allow patient-level analyses not always captured in quantitative population data. Metzl's ethnographic observations in *Dying of Whiteness* (2019a), along with interviews of family members and direct informants, complement numerical data analysis and policy reviews (e.g., Kalesan et al. 2017). In addition, insights from interviews can inform common ground between firearm safety advocates and gun rights activities. For example, in one interview by Metzl (2019a) of a relative who had recently completed a suicide with a firearm, the relative stated they were not anti-gun and still believed in protection of gun rights. However, that same relative suggested that it should be a criminal offense to have an unlocked gun in a house. In other interviews conducted by Metzl, support for background checks was voiced by multiple families who underwent trauma from relative suicide events.

NFGSW ETHNOGRAPHY

Laurence Ralph (2014) and John Rich (2009) have also offered important narrative accounts of NFGSW survivors. Ralph spent conducting participant observation among gang members and former gang members, leading to publication of Renegade Dreams (Ralph 2014). The book details structural risk for firearm violence (a neighborhood that seems to hold captive the residents while being ignored by the city for funding improvements) as well as the markers of entry into gang life. However, Ralph spends much of the book focusing on how NFGSW injuries transform lives and identities both medically and culturally by spending significant time with the Crippled Footprint Collective—a group of paralyzed ex-gang members who advocate and educate about the dangers of gang life. Essentially, these individuals are respectfully discharged from gang life and seen as providing the ultimate sacrifice, in some ways even more so than death as they are then encouraged and supported when moving on to talk about dangers of being in a gang. Ralph resolves this conflict of gang support for ex-gang members educating at-risk youth about the dangers of gang membership as recognition that these NFGSW survivors have given the highest valued offering—their bodies. While Ralph's work does not specifically focus on an intervention aimed at reducing firearm violence, or even explicitly state that as the goal of his work, the ethnographic account provides valuable cultural insight into why and how those who engage in peer-peer firearm violence arise at those decisions.

John Rich, a primary care physician who was initially working in Boston, spent hours interviewing other black men who had been injured by gunshot wounds. Rich's work (2011) details the cultural system that develops for inner city young people with little hope of a life outside of violence through their attempts to "be known" through the use of guns or through injury from a gun. Metzl (2019a), Ralph (2014) and Rich (2011) all offer important ethnographic insight into the lives of NFGSW survivors and disparate cultural aspects of firearm life (rural uneducated whites, gang members, and inner-city youth).

Public health strategies often rest on increasing education and access to a specific intervention or treatment strategy as means to decrease a specific outcome. Interventions focused on reducing gun-related morbidity and mortality will have to move beyond a singular public health approach and take into account the culturally based, symbolic lives of firearms. Metzl (2019a) has addressed this issue through his long-term ethnographic interviewing of mostly white male gun owners, as well as analysis of gun policy in different states and throughout the history of the United States. He examines the socio-political and cultural contexts surrounding firearms and specifically uncovers the "links between guns and larger scripts about identity, bias, racism, nationalism" (Metzl 2019b).

What do guns mean when they are not shooting bullets? Guns denote strong, culturally based feelings around protecting home and family, a sense of duty and conviction to make your community safer (Metzl 2019b). There is a disconnect between gun rights advocates and public health models focused on reducing firearm-related injuries through more restrictive gun buying and ownership policies. Gun owners see this as a tainted public health model that reduces gun ownership given that gun ownership is associated with duty, conviction and protecting? This disconnect introduces suspicion of bias toward medical groups and public health organizations (who bemoan the NRA led restrictions on public financing of firearm violence research that existed up until very recently). Metzl feels that firearm researchers do not help themselves when they fail to communicate with communities where gun ownership is common (2019b).

Metzl finds that for gun owners, guns are a form of selfhood, representing family heritage, bonds between neighbors, hobbies and activities and ways to bond with children. Taking those guns away takes away the family and those customs—that selfhood is robbed (Metzl 2019b). In themes common with Case and Deaton (2015, 2020), the changing economics of white mean—challenged by increasing opportunities for women, policies that end racism, real declines in wages when compared to college-educated individuals, we observe a remaining sense of identity that becomes increasingly critical to maintain.

As power tilts away from rural communities and less educated urban white areas, firearm ownership may create a way to "get back," by carrying guns to "instill fear particularly among urban and educated elites who hold the levers of power and status in society today" (Metzl 2019b). Also note the ability to code white man machismo into identity through imagined pasts of twentieth-century cowboy inventions of a non-existent nineteenth-century reality (Metzl allows those guns were an important aspect of American westward expansion but not in the John Wayne style way created for Hollywood movies). This leads to racialist thinking (consider a black man holding a gun compared to white man carrying one) of "white, good guys to protect against racial others" (e.g., carjackers, "thugs" vs. patriots, potential scenarios hinting at blackness instead of actual threats). While most medical conditions likely require more than a straightforward public health approach to decrease an undesired outcome, Metzl's social science approach demonstrates that most medical problems likely require more than education to move behavior given the deeply engrained cultural wiring of symbolic realities (Metzl 2019b).

MENTAL HEALTH, POPULATION HEALTH, AND NONFATAL GUNSHOT WOUND RESEARCH

The past three decades of gun safety research has coalesced around several important themes that will drive the future of gun safety research. First mental health is an important issue in the public health of the United States but is likely a separate issue from gun safety. Instead, differences in firearm mortality rates, including suicide and homicide, are best explained by differences in laws and policies relegating access to firearms. Second, while public health, quantitative and population level analyses are certainly important for identifying large scale trends and patterns in firearm safety data, patient level, ethnographic and qualitative data is needed to further refine hypotheses and to craft best approaches toward potential interventions aimed at reducing firearm-related mortality. Social science approaches to gun safety help show different issues related to gun ownership for different populations—that is, minorities (Rich 2011, Ralph 2014) and mainstream populations. Social science can also inform the cultural meanings around firearms while also identifying common ground across seemingly disparate political groups. Finally, the emotional, physical and financial cost of NFGSWs is large. Victims of NFGSW also are at increased risk for firearm mortality. Further work with patients that have experienced a recent or past NFGSW may inform future public health interventions aimed at reducing gun violence by creating distributions of potential issues directly from those most at risk that have undergone the outcome of concern.

OUR NFGSW STUDY

In 2019, we initiated a mixed methods project at an urban ED as part of the Research in Patient-Physician Interaction (chapter 3) course that the co-authors have co-taught each year. The motivation for this came from our understanding of the importance of firsthand interviewing of NFGSW injury patients and our unique position to be able to conduct firearm-related research without federal funding. The mass shooting in Las Vegas (2018) had just occurred as we planned our spring 2019 course. More specifically, Baer questioned whether the class could do something to address the issue of firearm injuries. The question was, "Could students interview patients with gunshot wounds who presented to the ED?" Wilson noted that while some of these patients came in through the trauma bay and were excluded from all of our studies, many waited in the waiting room, as did other patients with non-life-threatening and nonfatal injuries. And patients who came in through the trauma section of the ED were often hospitalized for several days after their condition was stabilized. This led to the creation of our study on NFGSWs.

We designed a study that could be undertaken by each successive cohort of undergraduate students in the patient-physician interaction course, with the goal to fill this gap in academic literature regarding the experiences of NFGSW survivors. While there have been reports of the experiences of individual patients who have survived firearm injuries (Kalra 2019, Rich 2011, Ralph 2007), the literature is lacking in studies of the social, physiological, financial, and emotional impact of such injuries in a larger group of patients. Nor are there such studies of the symbolic meanings of firearms to those who own them (Metzl 2019b). We actually know very little about these issues for survivors of NFGSW injuries (Bernstein 2017). In addition, other first-hand narratives, ethnographies, and interviews have come from community participation, and no studies have been conducted in clinical settings. The ED is an ideal field site in further examining the experiences of patients most affected by these types of traumatic events. The ED is additionally an optimal site at gaging how the gun violence epidemic is manifesting within the major communities serviced by an urban ED in the U.S. southeast.

NFGSW STUDY METHODS

The aim of this study is to examine the unique experiences of patients involved in nonfatal gun violence events. Our goal is to investigate the perceptions of patients regarding safety, being involved in gun violence events, as well as any concerns brought up by study participants. Ideally, study results can be used to inform potential changes and interventions aimed at decreasing firearm violence via patient-informed approaches.

Initially, the study was designed to only enroll and interview patients who had been shot. However, this study was also part of a student class project and, during that semester, an unseasonable cold snap seemed to lead to fewer shootings than expected. Thus, we expanded to include a control group of males (since most of our GSW victims in the ED are male) who had not been shot. Overall, we have a control group of non-gun violence patients and two groups of participants that have been shot: a NFGSW group of acutely injured patients and a group of patients who have previously experiences gunshot wounds.

The guiding research questions for this study were: What are the experiences of patients involved in nonfatal gun violence events? How do the experiences of these patients defer from those of patients who have never been involved with nonfatal gun violence events?

The study employs a cross-sectional design and qualitative approach using semi-structured interviews to gain insight into the downstream impacts of NFGSWs. The study was reviewed by the University of South Florida IRB (Pro00034945) and it was approved to include the use of verbal informed consent using a study script with patients who meet inclusion criteria. The data is deidentified after verbal consent is obtained (i.e., we only use identifiers to pre-screen patients utilizing the electronic medical record in the ED).

RESULTS

At the time of this writing, we had interviewed approximately 50 participants who had not been involved in gun violence and have closed enrollment of that arm as of summer 2021. We are still enrolling adult patients who have recently been shot or shot in the past. Seventy-seven participants with a prior gunshot wound have been interviewed as of June 2020. As of July 2020, this study is ongoing, so here we present a snapshot of some of the results to date. In this summary interim snapshot, we focus on the responses of the gunshot wound patients (GSW N = 13, 13 male) and previous gunshot wound patients (PGSW N = 17, 14 male, 3 female). We have chosen to compare these two groups as we feel there is urgency around capturing the voices of those who have survived NFGSW injuries and also wanted to see if perspectives change after survivors are forced to deal with downstream sequelae of their wounds over long periods of time.

Most participants who had recently been shot were young. Seventy-seven of the participants were under 40 and half of the participants were under 30 years old. In comparison, many of our participants who had previously been injured in the remote past were over the age of 50 (49%) and one-fourth of those participants were even over the age of 60. Our early data collection did not include specific information regarding how long ago patients had previously been shot. However, we suspect that the time period is likely 20 to 25 years ago given the data we have collected for acute gunshot wound injuries. We have now added specific questions regarding how long ago participants have been shot to better understand the number of life—years represented by people living with prior gunshot wounds, as well as the potential effects of perspective years after an initial injury.

We know from epidemiological data that white males represent large numbers of gunshot wound fatalities by suicide. Thus, it was not surprising that the majority of our prior and acute gunshot wound patients are Black (over 55%) or Hispanic (25%). Many of the patients that had been shot previously were still presenting to the ED with pain-related complaints that they traced, at least partially back to the index gunshot wound event.

FIREARM OWNERSHIP

"If you are not crazy, do what you like."—32-year-old African American Male, acute gunshot wound participant on his views regarding handgun ownership.

Gun ownership was about the same for those in the ED after acute gun injuries (31% admitted to owning guns) compared to prior gunshot wound injured patients (35% admitted to currently owning a firearm). However, the percent of prior gunshot wound injured patients who used to own a gun but no longer do so was 18%, compared to only 1% in the acute injury group. In addition, the percent of participants who felt that everyone should be able to own guns was much higher in the acute GSW group (46%), compared to the previous GSW group, where participants felt more strongly that people with prior criminal convictions and mental illness should be excluded from gun ownership. Only 29% of patients with prior GSW injuries felt that everyone should be able to own a gun. One African American male who had recently been shot responded with a similar position emphasizing guns and protection: "Anyone [should be able to own a gun], as long as it's for protection." A white male who been shot previously, still supported broad gun ownership rights: "Everyone [should be able to own a gun], let Darwin decide." The majority of respondents in both groups felt that handguns or hunting rifles should be legal, but there was a noticeable drop in support for gun ownership years after a prior gunshot wound injury (54% prior gunshot wound group and 71% gunshot wound group). Of note, while most acute and previous NFGSW participants supported legal handgun and hunting rifle ownership, the majority did think that firearms such as the AR-15 should be legal. 54% of acute GSW participants did not think "assault" rifles should be legal, while 76% of previous GSW participants did not support keeping these types of firearms legal.

Many respondents in this limited sample analysis did not respond to questions about gun policy ("What should we do about guns in Florida?"). Representative answers from participants who did respond include the following:

> Guns aren't the issue—people are.—African American Male, 29 years old, GSW.
>
> Get rid of all of them.—African American Female, 44-year-old, PGSW.
>
> Nothing's going to change.—African American Male, 20 years old, GSW.
>
> Stronger regulations and no AR sales.—White Male, 37 years old, PGSW.

When asked if "things" would be better if there were no guns, most participants that were acutely injured disagreed with this statement (69%) while those that had previously been injured (and were older) agreed 47% of the time. Overall, the majority of patients did not feel that things would get better if there were no guns. Interestingly, while the majority of GSW responded no (69%), the PGSW patients were split with 47% each responding yes and no.

Would things be better if there were no guns?

> Yes. . . . It wouldn't be perfect.—African American Male, 73 years old, PGSW.
>
> No. [It] only takes one bad man to kill all these people in schools, but it only takes one good man with a gun to stop [them].—White Male, 61 years old, GSW.
>
> No. [We] need it for protection from animals and people.—African American Male, 22 years old, GSW.
>
> No. It would get worse. [There would be] more stabbing[s]. People are the problem.—African American Male, 27 years old, GSW.

CAUSES AND RESULTS OF INJURY

The most common reason for a gunshot wound was an act of interpersonal violence including an altercation/conflict, drive-by shooting, or robbery. This was reported in 38% of the firearm injuries among black and Hispanic participants. Many injuries also occurred by accident, usually when cleaning or showing a gun to others (31%).

HOW DID YOU GET SHOT?

Accidental:

> Didn't know [the gun] was loaded.—Hispanic Male, 29 years old, PGSW.
>
> I was negligent. I was putting together and putting apart a gun. . . . Did not take the proper precautions.—Hispanic Male, 20s, GSW.
>
> Leaving event, taking out my gun to put in the car and it shot me in the groin and into thigh.—Hispanic Male, 22 years old, GSW.
>
> At coworkers house, was being shown a gun. Friend went to clear the gun, discharged; hit the tile floor and ricocheted into my leg.—White Male, 21 years old, GSW.
>
> Shot myself in the hand; was lubricating the gun; was a new gun.—White Male, 52 years old, GSW

Got shot in hand at 13 years old. A kid was playing with a gun. I told him to stop playing with it and I reached my hand in his jacket and it went off.—Hispanic Male, 22 years old, PGSW.

Aggression from others:

Picking up a hitchhiker.—White Male, 49 years old, PGSW

Breaking up a fight.—African American Male, PGSW

Was shot when I woke up.—Hispanic Male, 22 years old, GSW

Standing outside of a night club. Was rolling a blunt. Cops drove by and I turned away. The bullet came from left side and hit my left calf.—African American Male, 20s, GSW

Just hanging out on 19th street trying to smoke, didn't know who the guy was. It was just the two of them out there.—African American Male, 27 years old, GSW

Guy walked on up to me, tried to rob me, [shot me], I ran to the store, and passed out.—African American Male, 37 years, GSW

10 years old with cousin at a party, cousin's boyfriend started fighting with her. There was a huge fight, got cornered at dead end, they started shooting. [Second was] 17 years old playing paintball, neighbor was hunting and the shot hit a tree like 10 feet away.—African American Male, 37 years old, PGSW

I was in the wrong place at the wrong time. I was just hanging out.—White Male PGSW

I got shot 6 times from the waist up by an AR-15.—Black Male, PGSW

Many participants were shot in the lower extremities—for example, leg or foot (54%). The most common issues facing those who had been shot were financial or related to disability and further medical issues, including pain management. One participant specifically mentioned PTSD that resulted from the injury:

Took two years to work again [after a] knee replacement.—African American Female, 51 years old, PGSW

I was just happy to be alive.—White Male, 66 years old, PGSW

I am no longer fully mobile.—Hispanic Male, 90 years old, GSW

I was supposed to play basketball for LSU on a scholarship.—White Male 24 GSW

Had stage 3 renal failure.—Hispanic Male, 90 years old, GSW

Hadn't thought about it, have been in jail for 13 years.—African American Male, 38 years old, GSW

With regard to what could be changed to prevent GSWs, responses included the following:

Make sure police technology that can better solve gun violence actually works.—Black Male, 43

Not be so stupid.—White Male, 53

I wouldn't have fought so hard to stay alive.—Black Male, 34

Stay away from guns.—Black Male, 62

Better healthcare system.—Black Male, 40

Now I do what I need to protect myself.—White Male, 37

Change the places you go, people you are with, and things you do.—Hispanic Male, 38

I'd try to make changes in how easy to get guns, especially for kids.—Black Male, 74 years old

I think there should be a cutoff point; if you're born after that date, you can't own guns.—White Male, 38 years old

People shouldn't have guns—African American Female, 51 years old, PGSW

Everyone should have a gun; nurses, teachers, everyone. This will prevent mass shootings.—African American male, 20s, GSW

Strict gun laws everywhere.—African American Male, 37 years old, GSW

Even if [someone is] on probation, [they should] be able to carry, but have a special way to handle it.—African American Male, 22 years old, GSW

How long does it take to get your rights back? You're telling me that because I have a felony, "I'm not allowed to protect my family?"—African American Male, 20

No, I still like them. I just wish I had a way to find out where mine is now.—African American Male, 34

Going to teach my kids how to shoot and self—defense. It has come down to shoot to live.—African American male, 34

Everything sucks from a wheelchair. . . . I was depressed for a year.—White Male, 49 years old, PGSW

Not a lot has changed. No long–term effects other than the job situation because I can't stand for too long or be harnessed like I used to.—White Male, 38 years old, PGSW

Police can't protect you all the time. Everyone should own guns.—African American Male, 20s, GSW

No[t] going to walk the same. [I] can't play with [my] kids. My kids have to see this.—African American Male, 37 years old, GSW

Stay in your own lane is the lesson. Dip and dive. Stay away from people. Keep to yourself. Keep family close. You never know who can cause problems.—African American Male, 27 years old, GSW

CONCLUSIONS AND THE ANTHROPOLOGICAL DIFFERENCE

Quantitative studies have investigated gunshot wound data at the population health level, and such analyses are critical for demonstrating that an epidemiological problem exists (Kalesan 2017). Specifically, attention has been paid to the fact that approximately 40,000 people a year die from firearms. This is devastating. However, most people survive firearm injuries, and the impact of those injuries may last be ongoing for many years. Those injured by firearms are often less than 30 years old with long lives of pain, financial impacts, lost job prospects, and more violence ahead of them. While other researchers have examined these survivors quantitatively (Ranney et al. 2017), others have also produced critical ethnographic material narrating the lives of participants with NFGSWs (e.g., Rich 2011; Richardson 2015; Ralph 2014).

We have presented our framework for ongoing research with NFGSW survivors; work is being done directly in the clinical space. Not only are we interviewing those who have been shot in the remote past, but also patients who have been shot recently. While the results presented here are preliminary, we already recognize a likely impact of time and perspective that seems to occur among cohorts of people who have been shot in the past. In our interim analysis, participants with prior gunshot wound injuries were more likely to support stricter firearm access laws and to limit the types of firearms available. Those patients also demonstrated insight into how their previous injuries had impacted their lives (continued pain, less job prospects, paralysis).

Our ultimate goal is to understand the structural and cultural issues involved in firearm injuries. Analyses of these primary data show a trend for minorities to be injured by others, due to the structural issues in their neighborhoods. The pattern follows the ethnographic data of Rich (2011) and Ralph (2014). Patients from the majority population were more likely to injure themselves while interacting with their firearm, suggesting a pattern related to symbolic and cultural issues related to guns, following the patterns Metzl (2019a) has discussed.

We are continuing to build on our data set. The anthropological difference—the qualitative method we utilize, enables us to see differences in populations impacted by firearm violence, as well as the structural and cultural issues related to these injuries. The insights will not only be important for better understanding of NFGSW injuries but also, ideally, will also be utilized to inform potential change and interventions to address the complex causes of these injuries. We feel that the way to find ways to decrease future firearm violence is by better understanding the lives and perspectives of those who suffer these injuries.

Conclusion

In this book we have illustrated what we feel is a useful approach to a critical, clinically applied medical anthropology. Certainly, it is not easy to access medical settings, such as the Emergency Department of a major urban hospital. But it can be done. And, we have seen that as word of our projects has spread, the medical system has reached out to offer us increased access.

We feel that our work is firmly grounded in the history and theory of medical anthropology, a kind of "back to the future." We also feel that our work shows another possibility for employment of medical anthropologists, a key contemporary concern. In addition, the work introduced here demonstrates ways to improve the patient experience by integrating key components of anthropology into medical education. We believe that a multifaceted approach of having medical anthropologists integrated directly into clinical healthcare teams, along with blending the education of anthropology graduate students and medical students/residents, and, specifically designing a structural curriculum for physician education, will, together, lead to a shift in the clinical gaze in medicine over a long period of time, and open up new pathways for patient care previously unimagined.

The ongoing paradigm shift toward value-based care in medicine is opening doors for new members of interdisciplinary care teams. Physicians, medical social workers, and case managers cannot do it all. Patient experience has become a key part of medical reimbursement and all medical facilities have offices of patient experience. Who better to staff such offices than medical anthropologists who have had experience as students in clinical settings? In addition, as quality care and improved outcomes are emphasized for vulnerable populations and diagnoses (e.g., those with sickle cell disease), the ability for medical anthropologists to identify social, cultural, economic, and medical connections, as well as connections and networks across communities of people, becomes invaluable contributions.

CLINICAL ANTHROPOLOGY 2.0

We feel that what we have presented here is a new approach to clinically applied anthropology (Chrisman 1982) which is not subservient to biomedicine, but rather which trains biomedical personnel to effect changes in the way the system functions, at least in terms of the patient experience. We are also reclaiming applied anthropological work (Rylko-Bauer et al., 2006). This approach integrates the strengths of cultural, structural, and critical theory in order to solve problems directly in clinical spaces—not to just play role as observer of the biomedical system. The separation between theory and praxis is an artificial separation that we move past, utilizing and developing anthropological theory while finding applications that help patients, physicians, and healthcare systems solve real problems that, without anthropology, are reified and reproduced during each clinical encounter. Our methods grow out of classical anthropological theory and methods. We hope that by training the actors in the system in a different fashion, they will be positioned and motivated to make further changes in the overall system.

IMPLICATIONS OF THIS WORK: EDUCATION

Future work should continue to formally introduce patient-centered perspectives, the role of culture, and the role of structure of premedical and medical students to postgraduate medical residents, practicing physicians, and healthcare administrators. The patient experience, value-based care, and quality outcomes will continue to grow in importance, but often lead to frustration, and are treated as an afterthought in the current curriculum. Our approach, instead, integrates an anthropological perspective at different points in the curriculum to, over time, shift and integrate the view of clinical administrators and medical practitioners in an attempt to close the gap between the explanatory models presented by Kleinman et al., over 40 years ago. The cultures and explanatory models of healthcare providers and of patients are still distinct. Specifically, we feel strongly that patient shadowing, essentially the same thing as participant observation, is a key technique that, even in a short amount of time, can drastically alter the clinical gaze of even experienced healthcare system workers. It serves to sensitize them to the experience of the patient.

In addition, our education model places anthropology graduate students into clinical spaces, learning what problems are relevant, why patients suffer, and how they might be able to work with physicians and healthcare systems to solve clinical problems. This model of education in anthropology opens up new job opportunities for medical anthropologists and gives medical anthropology interdisciplinary relevance and visibility.

IMPLICATIONS OF THIS WORK: CLINICAL

The goal of our projects is not to solely comment, critique, and observe. Instead, our approach has been to find places of suffering and stagnation—problems that do not have an obvious answer, or where the solutions have led to unacceptable outcomes, for both providers and patients. Often this approach means first conducting participant observation, interviews with participants (patients, physicians, administrators), and creating ethnographies to then drive hypotheses for approaches to change (leaflets, opioid pathways, sickle cell pain management). We believe that this patient-centered ethnographic approach will highlight unseen clinical problems and open up pathways of treatment that were previously unseen to nonanthropologists. Our work has led to direct improvements in medical outcomes (e.g., treatment of opioid use disorder and hepatitis C) as well as improved the patient experience during the clinical encounter (leaflet, translation services, communication).

IMPLICATIONS OF THIS WORK: PUBLIC HEALTH

The nonfatal gunshot wound project hints at new ways to address long-standing public health emergencies. Multiple approaches have been attempted to decrease firearm-related violence, but the success of many public health attempts is not well understood (partially because public funding to study those attempts has been banned for so long). Our work with patients who have been injured by previous gunshots focuses on their lived experiences and generates data that highlight important areas of focus to those most affected by this violence. Ideally, this approach to public health will lead to patient-informed interventions—hypotheses for firearm violence reduction based on the experiences of patients themselves and aimed at what best might decrease future episodes of injury. Our data also point to at least two distinct populations with different cultural values and structural positions with regard to firearm injuries.

MOVING FORWARD

Old models of applied medical anthropology were generated in old ways of practicing medicine—namely where singe physician-patient encounters were most important and where the goal, for many physicians, was to increase patient compliance with specific care plans. Kleinman et al. (1978) and Hahn (1996) rightly demonstrated the difficulty in gaining improved "compliance" when the explanatory models between patients and providers were so far apart between illness and disease, and between the culture of patients and the culture of biomedicine. However, now, the problems in healthcare are much more complex than single patient encounters and medical compliance. In addition, the superficiality of earlier approaches used by clinically based anthropologists can be complemented and improved by integrating specific aspects of critical medical anthropology—particularly concepts of structural violence. This was over 40 years ago. Medicine and anthropology have evolved since the heyday of Clinically Applied Anthropology (CAA 1.0) 40 years ago. But the gaps in explanatory models, the suffering of patients, and dysfunction of the healthcare system continue, and have only become more complex.

There is growing recognition that physicians must manage not just the patient in front of them, but the reasons why the patient arrived in the situation that they did and how the experience of patients can be improved. To get there, integration of social domains of medicine and patient-centered approaches are important, but education curriculum is still nascent in designing that integration into current training. As a result of this failure of training, physicians become frustrated and burned out when their satisfaction scores remain flat and so much is asked of them not just for the treatment of specific patients but also for the growing role to help improve healthcare systems.

Now is an interdisciplinary moment in medicine, the recognition that physicians cannot fix anything alone. This moment allows for medical anthropologists to add value to these healthcare teams delivering complex care. The specific way those medical anthropologists can be utilized is in the improvement of the patient experience, the creation of patient-centered interventions and new clinical pathway development, as well as ideas for improving public health. Anthropologists can contribute to the directions necessary for training of contemporary physicians. And the opening for medical anthropologists to work with healthcare teams also provides special access to vulnerable patient populations that have been hard to reach for social scientists—for example, those in acute opioid withdrawal, those with acute sickle cell pain crisis, and those who have been shot. IRB permission to work with such populations is challenging. However, working with the medical system, allows anthropologists the opportunity to engage in Quality Improvement projects, gaining access, and having the opportunity to discover and implement real change for these patients and to these systems. Those ethnographies, participant observation, interviews, and use of other anthropological methods can also lead to important contributions to the medical as well as public health literature, informing for patient-centered interventions (e.g., GSW). The role of medical anthropologists in the clinical space is not subservient to biomedicine but, instead, offers new ways to advance anthropological theory and praxis, to critique, but also to actually solve, problems. Applied anthropologists discovered years ago that the only way to effect change was to be in the positions where decisions were being made. We call for the same approach to be used in the clinical and public health realms. If we are inside the system, we gain the power to implement real change. Now is the time for us to synthesize the approaches into a Clinical Anthropology 2.0.

References

18 HIPAA identifiers: Information technology services: Loyola university Chicago. (n.d.). Retrieved June 18, 2021, from Luc.edu website: https://www.luc.edu/its/aboutits/itspoliciesguidelines/hipaainformation/18hipaaidentifiers

2016 Cleveland Clinic's latest initiative: Shadowing patients to improve their experience. (2016). *Advisory Board—the Daily Briefing*. Retrieved from https://www.advisory.com/daily-briefing/2016/01/08/shadowing-patients-to-improve-their-experience

ACEP. (2015). Acute Unscheduled Care Model (AUCM): Enhancing Appropriate Admissions A Physician-Focused Payment Model (PFPM) for Emergency Medicine. Retrieved June 28, 2021, from HHS website: https://aspe.hhs.gov/system/files/pdf/255906/ProposalACEP.pdf

Adams, V., Burke, N. J., & Whitmarsh, I. (2014). Slow research: Thoughts for a movement in global health. *Medical Anthropology*, *33*(3), 179–197.

Agamben, G. (1999). *Homo Sacer: Sovereign Power and Bare Life*. Pre-Textos.

Aisiku, I. P., Smith, W. R., McClish, D. K., Levenson, J. L., Penberthy, L. T., Roseff, S. D., … Roberts, J. D. (2009). Comparisons of high versus low emergency department utilizers in sickle cell disease. *Annals of Emergency Medicine*, *53*(5), 587–593.

American foundation for firearm injury reduction in medicine. (n.d.). Retrieved July 9, 2021, from Affirmresearch.org website: https://affirmresearch.org/

APM Gun Survey, Part One: "Red flag" laws — APM Research Lab. (2019, August 20). Retrieved July 9, 2021, from Apmresearchlab.org website: https://www.apmresearchlab.org/gun-survey-red-flag

BirdStrike, Zachman MD MPH, S., Emily D'Amelio, R. N., Grinspoon, P., Adelman, S., Woroniecka, K., … Fery Pashang, P. (2013, November 19). The focus on patient satisfaction is enough to make you sick. Retrieved June 30, 2021, from Kevinmd.com website: https://www.kevinmd.com/blog/2013/11/focus-patient-satisfaction-sick.html

Bliley, T. (2000). *Drug Addiction Treatment Act of 2000*.

Bodenheimer, T., & Sinsky, C. (2014). From triple to quadruple aim: Care of the patient requires care of the provider. *Annals of Family Medicine*, *12*(6), 573–576.

Body, R., Kaide, E., Kendal, S., & Foex, B. (2015). Not all suffering is pain: Sources of patients' suffering in the emergency department call for improvements in communication from practitioners. *Emergency Medicine Journal: EMJ*, *32*(1), 15–20.

Branson, B. M., Handsfield, H. H., Lampe, M. A., Janssen, R. S., Taylor, A. W., Lyss, S. B., … Centers for Disease Control and Prevention (CDC). (2006). Revised recommendations for HIV testing of adults, adolescents, and pregnant women in health-care settings. *Recommendations and Reports: Morbidity and Mortality Weekly Report*, *55*(RR-14), 1–17; quiz CE1-4.

Brenner, J. (2014, March 7). Camden Hot Spotting Trial Protocol. Retrieved June 26, 2021, from Nejm.org website: https://www.nejm.org/doi/suppl/10.1056/NEJMsa1906848/suppl_file/nejmsa1906848_protocol.pdf

Bronsky, E. S., McGraw, C., Johnson, R., Giordano, K., Orlando, A., & Bar-Or, D. (2017). CARES: A community-wide collaboration identifies super-utilizers and reduces their 9-1-1 call, emergency department, and hospital visit rates. *Prehospital Emergency Care: Official Journal of the National Association of EMS Physicians and the National Association of State EMS Directors*, *21*(6), 693–699.

Bryk, J., Fischer, G. S., Lyons, A., Shroff, S., Bui, T., Simak, D., & Kapoor, W. (2018). Improvement in quality metrics by the UPMC enhanced care program: A novel super-utilizer program. *Population Health Management*, *21*(3), 217–221.

BUPE. (2021). Retrieved July 7, 2021, from Acep.org website: https://www.acep.org/patient-care/bupe/

Butkus, R., Doherty, R., Bornstein, S. S., & Health and Public Policy Committee of the American College of Physicians. (2018). Reducing firearm injuries and deaths in the United States: A position paper from the American College of Physicians. *Annals of Internal Medicine*, *169*(10), 704–707.

Carter, P. M., Walton, M. A., Roehler, D. R., Goldstick, J., Zimmerman, M. A., Blow, F. C., & Cunningham, R. M. (2015). Firearm violence among high-risk emergency department youth after an assault injury. *Pediatrics*, *135*(5), 805–815.

Case, A., & Deaton, A. (2015). Rising morbidity and mortality in midlife among white non-Hispanic Americans in the 21st century. *Proceedings of the National Academy of Sciences of the United States of America*, *112*(49), 15078–15083.

Case, A., & Deaton, A. (2020). *Deaths of Despair and the Future of Capitalism*. Princeton, NJ: Princeton University Press.

Chapman, S., Alpers, P., & Jones, M. (2016). Association between gun law reforms and intentional firearm deaths in Australia, 1979-2013. *JAMA: The Journal of the American Medical Association*, *316*(3), 291–299.

CHEO WELCOME TO OUR EMERGENCY DEPARTMENT. (2019, May). Retrieved July 6, 2021, from Cheo.on.ca website: https://www.cheo.on.ca/en/resources-and-support/resources/P5043E.pdf

Chicago Tribune. (2017, August 21). Tracking Chicago shooting victims: 2,021 so far this year, 164 more than in 2020. *Chicago Tribune*. Retrieved from https://www.chicagotribune.com/data/ct-shooting-victims-map-charts-htmlstory.html

Chrisman, N. J., Maretzki, T., & Maretzki, W. (Eds.). (1982). *Clinically Applied Anthropology: Anthropologists in Health Science Settings*. Dordrecht, Netherlands: Kluwer Academic.

Chrisman, N., Strickland, C., Powell, K., Squeochs, M., & Yallup, M. (1999). Community partnership research with the Yakama Indian nation. *Human Organization*, *58*(2), 134–141.

Clinician Resilience and Well-Being - National Academy of Medicine. (2016, October 4). Retrieved July 6, 2021, from Nam.edu website: https://nam.edu/initiatives/clinician-resilience-and-well-being/

CMS' Value-Based Programs. (n.d.). Retrieved June 1, 2021, from Cms.gov website: https://www.cms.gov/Medicare/Quality-Initiatives-Patient-Assessment-Instruments/Value-Based-Programs/Value-Based-Programs

Cordoba-Perez, A. (2020). *First-Ever Needle Exchange Program in Hillsborough County Approved by Commissioners*. Tampa: WUSF Public Media.

Crane, J., & Angrosino, M. (1992). *Field Projects in Anthropology. A Student Handbook. Chapter 5*. Long Grove, IL: Waveland Press.

Crossman, K. L., Wiener, E., Roosevelt, G., Bajaj, L., & Hampers, L. C. (2010). Interpreters: Telephonic, in-person interpretation and bilingual providers. *Pediatrics*, *125*(3), e631–e638.

Cultural Competency Training. (n.d.). Retrieved June 28, 2021, from Cigna.com website: https://www.cigna.com/health-care-providers/resources/cultural-competency-training

Cunningham, E. B., Amin, J., Feld, J. J., Bruneau, J., Dalgard, O., Powis, J., … SIMPLIFY study group. (2018). Adherence to sofosbuvir and velpatasvir among people with chronic HCV infection and recent injection drug use: The SIMPLIFY study. *The International Journal on Drug Policy*, *62*, 14–23.

Curtin, S. C., Warner, M., & Hedegaard, H. (2016). Increase in suicide in the United States, 1999–2014. *NCHS Data Brief*, (241), 1–8. PMID: 27111185.

CyraCom. (2016, November 4). Retrieved June 30, 2021, from Cyracom.com website: https://interpret.cyracom.com/

Dempsey, C. (2017). *The Antidote to Suffering: How Compassionate Connected Care can Improve Safety, Quality, and Experience*. Columbus, OH: McGraw-Hill Education.

Diamond, L. C., Schenker, Y., Curry, L., Bradley, E. H., & Fernandez, A. (2009). Getting by: Underuse of interpreters by resident physicians. *Journal of General Internal Medicine*, *24*(2), 256–262.

D'Onofrio, G., O'Connor, P. G., Pantalon, M. V., Chawarski, M. C., Busch, S. H., Owens, P. H., … Fiellin, D. A. (2015). Emergency department-initiated buprenorphine/naloxone treatment for opioid dependence: A randomized clinical trial: A randomized clinical trial. *JAMA: The Journal of the American Medical Association*, *313*(16), 1636–1644.

Dressler, W. W. (2017). *Culture and the Individual: Theory and Method of Cultural Consonance*. Walnut Creek, CA: Left Coast Press.

Dzau, Victor J., Kirch, D. G., & Nasca, T. J. (2018). To care is human — Collectively confronting the clinician-burnout crisis. *The New England Journal of Medicine*, *378*(4), 312–314.

Emergency Department – St. Thomas Elgin General Hospital. (n.d.). Retrieved July 6, 2021, from Stegh.on.ca website: https://www.stegh.on.ca/hospital-services/emergency-department/

Emergency Medical Treatment & Labor Act (EMTALA). (n.d.). Retrieved June 28, 2021, from Cms.gov website: https://www.cms.gov/Regulations-and-Guidance/Legislation/EMTALA

Emergency narcotic addiction treatment. (n.d.). Retrieved July 7, 2021, from Usdoj.gov website: https://www.deadiversion.usdoj.gov/pubs/advisories/emerg_treat.htm

Ervin, A. M. (2000). *Applied Anthropology: Tools and Perspectives for Contemporary Practice*. Upper Saddle River, NJ: Pearson.

Erwin, D. (2008). The Witness Project. In J. McMullin & D. Weiner (Eds.), *Confronting Cancer* (pp. 125–146). Santa Fe: School for Advanced Research Press.

Farmer, P. (2003). *Pathologies of Power: Health, Human Rights, and the New War on the Poor*. Berkeley, CA: University of California Press.

Farmer, P. E., Nizeye, B., Stulac, S., & Keshavjee, S. (2006). Structural violence and clinical medicine. *PLoS Medicine*, *3*(10), e449.

Finkelstein, A., Zhou, A., Taubman, S., & Doyle, J. (2020). Health care hotspotting - A randomized, controlled trial. *The New England Journal of Medicine*, *382*(2), 152–162.

Fleming, M. D., Shim, J. K., Yen, I. H., Thompson-Lastad, A., Rubin, S., Van Natta, M., & Burke, N. J. (2017). Patient engagement at the margins: Health care providers' assessments of engagement and the structural determinants of health in the safety-net. *Social Science & Medicine (1982)*, *183*, 11–18.

Flores, G., Abreu, M., Barone, C. P., Bachur, R., & Lin, H. (2012). Errors of medical interpretation and their potential clinical consequences: A comparison of professional versus ad hoc versus no interpreters. *Annals of Emergency Medicine*, *60*(5), 545–553.

Florida Department of Health. (2017). Florida Health Community Health Assessment Resource Tool Set (CHARTS). Retrieved June 30, 2021, from http:// www .flhealthcharts.com/charts/default.aspx

Forde, C. A. (2014). *Emergency Medicine Triage as the Intersection of Storytelling, Decision-Making, and Dramaturgy*. University of South Florida.

Foucault, M. (1973). *The Birth of the Clinic: An Archaeology of Medical Perception*. New York: Pantheon Book.

Fox, J. A., & Fridel, E. E. (2016). The tenuous connections involving mass shootings, mental illness, and gun laws. *Violence and Gender*, *3*(1), 14–19.

Galtung, J. (1969). Violence, peace, and peace research. *Journal of Peace Research*, *6*(3), 167–191.

Garthwaite, Craig. (2019). All Medicaid Expansions Are Not Created Equal: The Geography and Targeting of the Affordable Care Act. Retrieved June 19, 2021, from Brookings.edu website: https://www.brookings.edu/wp-content/uploads/2019/09/Garthwaite-et-al_conference-draft.pdf

Gawande, A. (2011). The hot spotters: Can we lower medical costs by giving the neediest patients better care? *New Yorker (New York, N.Y.: 1925)*, 40–51.

Geertz, C. (1998, October 22). Deep hanging out. Retrieved June 18, 2021, from Nybooks.com website: https://www.nybooks.com/articles/1998/10/22/deep-hanging-out/

Gentilello, L. M., Rivara, F. P., Donovan, D. M., Jurkovich, G. J., Daranciang, E., Dunn, C. W., … Ries, R. R. (1999). Alcohol interventions in a trauma center as a means of reducing the risk of injury recurrence. *Annals of Surgery*, *230*(4), 473–480; discussion 480-3.

Ghany, M. G., Morgan, T. R., & AASLD-IDSA Hepatitis C Guidance Panel. (2020). Hepatitis C guidance 2019 update: American association for the study of liver diseases-infectious diseases society of America recommendations for testing, managing, and treating hepatitis C virus infection. *Hepatology (Baltimore, Md.)*, *71*(2), 686–721.

Gifford Medical Center Emergency Department, Randolph, VT: 24/7 emergency care. (n.d.). Retrieved July 6, 2021, from Giffordhealthcare.org website: https://giffordhealthcare.org/service/emergency-department/

Gifford's law center's annual gun law scorecard. (n.d.). Retrieved July 9, 2021, from Giffords.org website: https://giffords.org/lawcenter/resources/scorecard/

Goldstein, P. A., Storey-Johnson, C., & Beck, S. (2014). Facilitating the initiation of the physician's professional identity: Cornell's urban semester program. *Perspectives on Medical Education*, *3*(6), 492–499.

Good, B. J. (1992). *Lewis Henry Morgan Lectures: Medicine, Rationality and Experience: An Anthropological Perspective: An Anthropological Perspective.* doi: 10.1017/cbo9780511811029

Gravlee, C. C. (2009). How race becomes biology: embodiment of social inequality. *American Journal of Physical Anthropology*, *139*(1), 47–57.

Grebely, J., Dalgard, O., Conway, B., Cunningham, E. B., Bruggmann, P., Hajarizadeh, B., … SIMPLIFY Study Group. (2018). Sofosbuvir and velpatasvir for hepatitis C virus infection in people with recent injection drug use (SIMPLIFY): An open-label, single-arm, phase 4, multicentre trial. *The Lancet. Gastroenterology & Hepatology*, *3*(3), 153–161.

Grinshteyn, E., & Hemenway, D. (2019). Violent death rates in the US compared to those of the other high-income countries, 2015. *Preventive Medicine*, *123*, 20–26.

GroupMe Group text messaging with GroupMe. (2011). Retrieved June 18, 2021, from Groupme.com website: https://groupme.com/en-US/

Guidance Documents: QI, Research, Program Evaluation, Class/Student Project. (2015, November 1). Retrieved July 6, 2021, from BullsIRB website: https://irb.research.usf.edu/IRB/sd/Rooms/DisplayPages/LayoutInitial?Container=com.webridge.entity.Entity%5BOID%5BF648D6FB8E6911EA23A843A6163A0D00%5D%5D

Guns & Suicide. (2016, August 16). Retrieved July 9, 2021, from Harvard.edu website: https://www.hsph.harvard.edu/magazine/magazine_article/guns-suicide/

Hahn, R. A. (1996). *Sickness and Healing: An Anthropological Perspective.* New Haven, CT: Yale University Press.

Hansen, H., & Metzl, J. (2016). Structural competency in the U. S. healthcare crisis: Putting social and policy interventions into clinical practice. *Journal of Bioethical Inquiry*, *13*(2), 179–183.

Harvard Injury Control Research Center. (2011). The Australian Gun Buyback. Retrieved July 9, 2021, from BULLETins: Firearms research summaries website:

https://cdn1.sph.harvard.edu/wp-content/uploads/sites/1264/2012/10/bulletins_australia_spring_2011.pdf

HCAHPS: Patients' perspectives of care survey. (n.d.). Retrieved June 18, 2021, from Cms.gov website: https://www.cms.gov/Medicare/Quality-Initiatives-Patient-Assessment-Instruments/HospitalQualityInits/HospitalHCAHPS

Health Statistics - OECD. (n.d.). Retrieved June 19, 2021, from Oecd.org website: https://www.oecd.org/health/health-statistics.htm

Hein, I. (2019, December 5). "get out of the way DEA," physicians bid to treat addiction. Retrieved June 2, 2021, from Medscape website: https://www.medscape.com/viewarticle/922187

Hemmings, C. P. (2010). Rethinking medical anthropology: How anthropology is failing medicine. *Anthropology & Medicine*, *12*(2), 91–103.

Henderson, H. (2018). *"I am More Than my Addiction": Perceptions of Stigma and Access to Care in Acute Opioid Crisis* (University of South Florida, Tampa, Florida). Retrieved from https://scholarcommons.usf.edu/etd/7167/

Henderson, H. D. (2018). *"I am More than my Addiction": Perceptions of Stigma and Access to Care in Acute Opioid Crisis*. Graduate Theses and Dissertations. https://digitalcommons.usf.edu/etd/7167

Hoffman, J., & Tavernise, S. (2016, August 5). Vexing question on patient surveys: Did we ease your pain? *The New York Times*. Retrieved from https://www.nytimes.com/2016/08/05/health/pain-treatment-hospitals-emergency-rooms-surveys.html

Holmes, S. F. F., & Bodies, B. (2013). *Migrant Farmworkers in the United States*. Berkeley, CA: University of California Press.

Home: Society for applied anthropology. (n.d.). Retrieved July 5, 2021, from Appliedanthro.org website: http://appliedanthro.org

How do health expenditures vary across the population? (2019a, January 16). Retrieved June 19, 2021, from Kff.org website: https://www.kff.org/slideshow/how-health-expenditures-vary-across-the-population-slideshow/

How do health expenditures vary across the population? (2019b, January 16). Retrieved June 26, 2021, from Healthsystemtracker.org website: https://www.healthsystem-tracker.org/chart-collection/health-expenditures-vary-across-population/

How-to guide: Multidisciplinary rounds. (n.d.). Retrieved June 18, 2021, from Ihi.org website: http://www.ihi.org/resources/Pages/Tools/HowtoGuideMultidisciplinaryRounds.aspx

Human subjects research (HSR) | CITI program. (n.d.). Retrieved June 18, 2021, from CITI website: https://about.citiprogram.org/en/series/human-subjects-research-hsr/

Infectious Disease Elimination Act (IDEA). (n.d.). Retrieved July 3, 2021, from Floridahealth.gov website: http://www.floridahealth.gov/programs-and-services/idea/index.html

Interest Groups. (n.d.). Retrieved June 17, 2021, from Saem.org website: https://www.saem.org/about-saem/academies-interest-groups-affiliates2/join-an-interest-group

Jacobs, Z. G., Prasad, P. A., Fang, M. C., Abe-Jones, Y., & Kangelaris, K. N. (2019). The association between limited English proficiency and sepsis mortality. *Journal of Hospital Medicine: An Official Publication of the Society of Hospital Medicine*, *14*(Volume 15,03), E1–E7.

Jones, R. (2018, August 2). Death by patient satisfaction in the ER. Retrieved June 30, 2021, from Doximity.com website: https://www.doximity.com/articles/5aeb2380-aec7-431b-9ad5-c67c0ef21421?utm_campaign=identified_redirect&utm_source=opmed

Kalesan, B. (2017). The cost of firearm violence survivorship. *American Journal of Public Health*, *107*(5), 638–639.

Kellermann, A. L., Rivara, F. P., Rushforth, N. B., Banton, J. G., Reay, D. T., Francisco, J. T., … Somes, G. (1993). Gun ownership as a risk factor for homicide in the home. *The New England Journal of Medicine*, *329*(15), 1084–1091.

Kleinman, A. (1989). *The Illness Narratives: Suffering, Healing and the Human Condition*. London: Da Capo Press.

Kleinman, A., Eisenberg, L., & Good, B. (1978). Culture, illness, and care: Clinical lessons from anthropologic and cross-cultural research. *Annals of Internal Medicine*, *88*(2), 251–258.

Koop, C. E. (1992). Violence in America: A public health emergency: Time to bite the bullet back. *JAMA: The Journal of the American Medical Association*, *267* (22), 3075.

Krieger, N., Jahn, J. L., & Waterman, P. D. (2017). Jim Crow and estrogen-receptor-negative breast cancer: US-born black and white non-Hispanic women, 1992-2012. *Cancer Causes & Control: CCC*, *28*(1), 49–59.

Kristof, N. (2021, March 24). Opinion. *The New York Times*. Retrieved from https://www.nytimes.com/interactive/2017/11/06/opinion/how-to-reduce-shootings.html

Krogstad, J. M., Stepler, R., & Lopez, M. H. (2015, December 5). English proficiency on the rise among Latinos: U.S. born driving language changes. Retrieved June 30, 2021, from Pew Research Center website: https://www.pewhispanic.org/2015/05/12/english-proficiency-on-the-rise-among-latinos/

Language Services. (2016, November 10). Retrieved June 29, 2021, from Cyracom.com website: https://interpret.cyracom.com/services/

Larochelle, M. R., Bernson, D., Land, T., Stopka, T. J., Wang, N., Xuan, Z., … Walley, A. Y. (2018). Medication for opioid use disorder after nonfatal opioid overdose and association with mortality: A cohort study. *Annals of Internal Medicine*, *169*(3), 137–145.

Latour, B. (1993). *We Have Never Been Modern* (C. Porter, Trans.). London, England: Harvard University Press.

Leapfrog. (n.d.). Retrieved June 30, 2021, from Leapfroggroup.org website: https://www.leapfroggroup.org/

Lende, D. H., & Lachiondo, A. (2009). Embodiment and breast cancer among African American women. *Qualitative Health Research*, *19*(2), 216–228.

López, L., Rodriguez, F., Huerta, D., Soukup, J., & Hicks, L. (2015). Use of interpreters by physicians for hospitalized limited English proficient patients and its impact on patient outcomes. *Journal of General Internal Medicine*, *30*(6), 783–789.

Lyon-Callo, V. (2000). Medicalizing homelessness: The production of self-blame and self-governing within homeless shelters. *Medical Anthropology Quarterly*, *14*(3), 328–345.

Lyons, V. H., Rivara, F. P., Yan, A. N.-X., Currier, C., Ballsmith, E., Haggerty, K. P., … Rowhani-Rahbar, A. (2019). Firearm-related behaviors following firearm injury: Changes in ownership, carrying and storage. *Journal of Behavioral Medicine*, *42*(4), 658–673.

Madaras, L., Stonington, S., Seda, C. H., Garcia, D., & Zuroweste, E. (2019). Social distance and mobility - A 39-year-old pregnant migrant farmworker. *The New England Journal of Medicine*, *380*(12), 1093–1096.

Mancher, M., & Leshner, A. (2019). *Medications for Opioid Use Disorder Save Lives* (M. Mancher & A. Leshner, Eds.). Washington, DC: National Academies Press.

Mann, M. (2010). Pain, personhood, and translating sickle cell anemia1. *Transforming Anthropology*, *18*(2), 146–150.

Mater Emergency care. (n.d.). Retrieved July 6, 2021, from Mater Brisbane website: https://www.mater.org.au/health/services/emergency-care/emergency-care-public

Matthews, H. (2014). Cultural Broker or Collaborator? *Practicing Anthropology*, *36*(1), 16–20.

Mayo, R., Parker, V. G., Sherrill, W. W., Coltman, K., Hudson, M. F., Nichols, C. M., . . . Pribonic, A. P. (2016). Cutting corners: Provider perceptions of interpretation services and factors related to use of an ad hoc interpreter: Provider perceptions of interpretation services and factors related to use of an ad hoc interpreter. *Hispanic Health Care International: The Official Journal of the National Association of Hispanic Nurses*, *14*(2), 73–80.

McLellan, A. T., Lewis, D. C., O'Brien, C. P., & Kleber, H. D. (2000). Drug dependence, a chronic medical illness: Implications for treatment, insurance, and outcomes evaluation. *JAMA: The Journal of the American Medical Association*, *284*(13), 1689–1695.

Medicare Star Ratings. (n.d.). Retrieved July 5, 2021, from Medicare.gov website: https://www.medicare.gov/hospitalcompare/search.html

Merlino, J. (2014). *Service Fanatics: How to Build Superior Patient Experience the Cleveland Clinic Way*. New York, NY: McGraw-Hill Professional.

Metzl, J. M. (2018). Repeal the dickey amendment to address polarization surrounding firearms in the United States. *American Journal of Public Health*, *108*(7), 864–865.

Metzl, J. M. (2019a). *Dying of Whiteness: How the Politics of Racial Resentment is Killing America's Heartland*. London, England: Basic Books.

Metzl, J. M. (2019b). What guns mean: The symbolic lives of firearms. *Palgrave Communications*, *5*(1), 1–5. doi:10.1057/s41599-019-0240-y

Metzl, J. M., & Hansen, H. (2014). Structural competency: Theorizing a new medical engagement with stigma and inequality. *Social Science & Medicine (1982)*, *103*, 126–133.

Miller, M., & Hemenway, D. (2008). Guns and suicide in the United States. *The New England Journal of Medicine*, *359*(10), 989–991.

Miller, M., Hemenway, D., & Azrael, D. (2007). State-level homicide victimization rates in the US in relation to survey measures of household firearm ownership, 2001-2003. *Social Science & Medicine (1982)*, *64*(3), 656–664.

Miller, M., Hepburn, L., & Azrael, D. (2017). Firearm acquisition without background checks: Results of a national survey. *Annals of Internal Medicine, 166*(4), 233–239.

Nading, A. M. (2019). *Mosquito Trails: Ecology, Health, and the Politics of Entanglement.* Berkeley, CA: University of California Press. doi:10.1525/9780520958562.

Nairn, S., Whotton, E., Marshal, C., Roberts, M., & Swann, G. (2004). The patient experience in emergency departments: A review of the literature. *Accident and Emergency Nursing, 12*(3), 159–165.

Nappi, A. (2016, October). *Implementation of Patient-Controlled Analgesia Creates Consistent Patient Expectations With no Negative Impacts on Operational Metrics or Patient Experience. Abstract Control Number 837.* Las Vegas, Nevada: American College of Emergency Physicians, Scientific Assembly.

National Highway Traffic Safety Administration (NHTSA). DOT HS. (2010). *An Analysis of the Significant Decline in Motor Vehicle Traffic Fatalities in 2008.*

National Hospital Ambulatory Medical Care Survey: 2015 Emergency Department Summary Tables. (2015). Retrieved July 6, 2021, from Cdc.gov website: https://www.cdc.gov/nchs/data/nhamcs/web_tables/2015_ed_web_tables.pdf

National Inpatient Hospital Costs: The Most Expensive Conditions by Payer, 2017 #261. (n.d.). Retrieved June 26, 2021, from Ahrq.gov website: https://www.hcup-us.ahrq.gov/reports/statbriefs/sb261-Most-Expensive-Hospital-Conditions-2017.jsp

NHE Fact Sheet. (n.d.). Retrieved June 19, 2021, from Cms.gov website: https://www.cms.gov/Research-Statistics-Data-and-Systems/Statistics-Trends-and-Reports/NationalHealthExpendData/NHE-Fact-Sheet

NHLBI. (2014). Evidence-based management of sickle cell disease: Expert panel report. *Pediatrics, 134*(6), e1775–e1775.

Office for Human Research Protections. (2010, January 28). The Belmont Report. Retrieved June 18, 2021, from Hhs.gov website: https://www.hhs.gov/ohrp/regulations-and-policy/belmont-report/index.html

Office for Human Research Protections (OHRP). (2016, February 16). 45 CFR 46. Retrieved June 18, 2021, from Hhs.gov website: https://www.hhs.gov/ohrp/regulations-and-policy/regulations/45-cfr-46/index.html

Ortner, S. B. (1984). Theory in anthropology since the sixties. *Comparative Studies in Society and History, 26*(1), 126–126.

Ortner, S. B. (2016). Dark anthropology and its others: Theory since the eighties. *HAU: Journal of Ethnographic Theory, 6*(1), 47–73.

Osorio-Cruz, C. A. J. W. W. (2016a). *Mixed Methods Approach to a Sickle Cell Disease Pain Management Strategy in the ED.* Symposium by the Sea, Boca Raton, Florida.

Osorio-Cruz, C. A. J. W. W. (2016b). *Mixed Methods Approach to a Sickle Cell Disease Pain Management Strategy in the ED. Poster Presentation.* Symposium by the Sea. Boca Raton, Florida.

Osorno-Cruz, C., Nappi, A., & Wilson, J. W. (2017, August). *Implementation of Patient-Controlled Analgesia Protocol for Sickle Cell Patients Presenting with Acute Pain Crisis Creates Consistent Patient Expectations With no Negative*

Impacts on Operation Metrics and Patient Experience. Symposium by the Sea. Boca Raton, Florida.

Osorno-Cruz, C., & Wilson, J. W. (2018, April). *Understanding the Sickle-Cell Patient Experience and New Approaches to Pain Management (TH-160). Anthropology and Special Patient Populations*. Philadelphia, Pennsylvania: Society for Academic Anthropology.

Patient Resources. (n.d.). Retrieved July 6, 2021, from Andersonregional.org website: https://www.andersonregional.org/patients-visitors/patient-resources/

Pines, J. M., Lotrecchiano, G. R., Zocchi, M. S., Lazar, D., Leedekerken, J. B., Margolis, G. S., & Carr, B. G. (2016). A conceptual model for episodes of acute, unscheduled care. *Annals of Emergency Medicine*, *68*(4), 484-491.e3.

Press Ganey Associates. (n.d.). Retrieved June 1, 2021, from Pressganey.com website: http://www.pressganey.com

Press, I. (2006). *Patient Satisfaction: Understanding and Managing the Experience of Care* (2nd ed.). Chicago, IL: Health Administration Press.

Quet, M. (2018). Pharmaceutical capitalism and its logistics: Access to hepatitis C treatment. *Theory, Culture & Society*, *35*(2), 67–89.

Rabin, R. C. (2020, November 17). 'how did we not know?' gun owners confront a suicide epidemic. *The New York Times*. Retrieved from https://www.nytimes.com/2020/11/17/health/suicide-guns-prevention.html

Ralph, L. (2014). *Renegade Dreams: Living through Injury in Gangland Chicago*. Chicago, IL: University of Chicago Press.

Ranney, M. L., Betz, M. E., & Dark, C. (2019). #ThisIsOurLane - firearm safety as health care's highway. *The New England Journal of Medicine*, *380*(5), 405–407.

Ranney, M. L., Fletcher, J., Alter, H., Barsotti, C., Bebarta, V. S., Betz, M. E., … ACEP Technical Advisory Group on Firearm Injury Research, a Subcommittee of the ACEP Research Committee. (2017). A consensus-driven agenda for emergency medicine firearm injury prevention research. *Annals of Emergency Medicine*, *69*(2), 227–240.

Rich, J. A. (2011). *Wrong Place, Wrong Time: Trauma and Violence in the Lives of Young Black Men*. Baltimore, MD: Johns Hopkins University Press.

Richardson, J. B., Jr, St Vil, C., & Cooper, C. (2016). Who shot ya? How emergency departments can collect reliable police shooting data. *Journal of Urban Health: Bulletin of the New York Academy of Medicine*, *93 Suppl 1*(S1), 8–31.

Richardson, J. B., Jr, & Vil, C. S. (2016). 'Rolling dolo': Desistance from delinquency and negative peer relationships over the early adolescent life-course. *Ethnography*, *17*(1), 47–71.

Romney, A. K., Weller, S. C., & Batchelder, W. H. (1986). Culture as consensus: A theory of culture and informant accuracy. *American Anthropologist*, *88*(2), 313–338.

Roscoe, L. A., Eisenberg, E. M., & Forde, C. (2016). The role of patients' stories in emergency medicine triage. *Health Communication*, *31*(9), 1155–1164.

Rylko-Bauer, B., Singer, M., & VAN Willigen, J. (2006). Reclaiming applied anthropology: Its past, present, and future. *American Anthropologist*, *108*(1), 178–190.

Salhi, B. (2018). *Diagnosis Homeless: Emergency Department "Super-Utilizers" and Urban Poverty in Atlanta, Georgia*. Emory University: PhD Dissertation.

Salhi, B. A., White, M. H., Pitts, S. R., & Wright, D. W. (2018). Homelessness and emergency medicine: Furthering the conversation. *Academic Emergency Medicine: Official Journal of the Society for Academic Emergency Medicine*, *25*(5), 597.

Santos, J., Jones, S., Wakefield, D., Grady, J., & Andemariam, B. (2016). Patient controlled analgesia for adults with sickle cell disease awaiting admission from the emergency department. *Journal de La Societe Canadienne Pour Le Traitement de La Douleur [Pain Research & Management]*, *2016*, 3218186.

Scheper-Hughes, N. (1990). Three propositions for a critically applied medical anthropology. *Social Science & Medicine (1982)*, *30*(2), 189–197.

Seligman, R. (2014). *Possessing Spirits and Healing Selves: Embodiment and Transformation in an Afro-Brazilian Religion* (2014th ed.). New York, NY: Palgrave Macmillan.

Seligman, Rebecca. (2014). *Possessing Spirits and Healing Selves: Embodiment and Transformation in an Afro-Brazilian Religion* (2014th ed.). Basingstoke, England: Palgrave Macmillan.

Seymour, C. K., Griffin, C., Holmes, S. M., & Martinez, C. (2018). Structural differential - A 32-year-old man with persistent wrist pain. *The New England Journal of Medicine*, *379*(25), 2385–2388.

Shem, S. (1979). *The House of God*. London, UK: Bodley Head.

Sherman, L. W. (2001). Reducing gun violence: What works, what doesn't, what's promising. *Criminal Justice*, *1*(1), 11–25.

Shi, B. A. W., Mh, P., & Wright, D. W. (2018). Homelessness and Emergency Medicine: Furthering the Conversation. *Academic Emergency Medicine*, *25*(5), 597.

Siegel, M., Ross, C. S., & King, C., 3rd. (2013). The relationship between gun ownership and firearm homicide rates in the United States, 1981-2010. *American Journal of Public Health*, *103*(11), 2098–2105.

Silva, M., Genoff, M., Zaballa, A., Stabler, S. M., Gany, F., & Diamond, L. (2014). Interpreting in palliative care: A systematic review of the impact of interpreters on the delivery of palliative care services to cancer patients with limited English proficiency. *Journal of Clinical Oncology: Official Journal of the American Society of Clinical Oncology*, *32*(31_suppl), 123–123.

Singer, A. J., Thode, H. C., Jr, & Pines, J. M. (2019). US emergency department visits and hospital discharges among uninsured patients before and after implementation of the Affordable Care Act. *JAMA Network Open*, *2*(4), e192662.

Singer, M., & Baer, H. (1995). *Critical medical anthropology* (2nd ed.). Amityville, NY: Baywood Publishing Company.

Singer, M., Bulled, N., Ostrach, B., & Mendenhall, E. (2017). Syndemics and the biosocial conception of health. *Lancet*, *389*(10072), 941–950.

Singer, M., & Clair, S. (2003). Syndemics and public health: Reconceptualizing disease in bio-social context. *Medical Anthropology Quarterly*, *17*(4), 423–441.

Social Determinants in Health. (n.d.). Retrieved June 1, 2021, from Saem.org website: https://www.saem.org/about-saem/academies/adiemnew/resources/aced-it/social-determinants-in-health

Social emergency medicine / population health / social determinants of health. (n.d.). Retrieved July 5, 2021, from Saem.org website: https://www.saem.org/about-saem/academies-interest-groups-affiliates2/join-an-interest-group/social-emergency-medicine-and-population-health/social-emergency-medicine-population-health-social-determinants-of-health

Sonis, J. D., Aaronson, E. L., Lee, R. Y., Philpotts, L. L., & White, B. A. (2018). Emergency department patient experience: A systematic review of the literature: A systematic review of the literature. *Journal of Patient Experience*, *5*(2), 101–106.

Spicer, E. H. (1952). *Human Problems in Technological Change*. Nashville, TN: John Wiley & Sons.

Stark, D. E., & Shah, N. H. (2017). Funding and publication of research on gun violence and other leading causes of death. *JAMA: The Journal of the American Medical Association*, *317*(1), 84–85.

Stelfox, H. T., Gandhi, T. K., Orav, E. J., & Gustafson, M. L. (2005). The relation of patient satisfaction with complaints against physicians and malpractice lawsuits. *The American Journal of Medicine*, *118*(10), 1126–1133.

Stonington, S. D., Holmes, S. M., Hansen, H., Greene, J. A., Wailoo, K. A., Malina, D., … Marmot, M. G. (2018). Case studies in social medicine — attending to structural forces in clinical practice. *The New England Journal of Medicine*, *379*(20), 1958–1961.

Survey Instruments. (n.d.). Retrieved June 29, 2021, from Hcahpsonline.org website: https://hcahpsonline.org/en/survey-instruments/

Federal Bureau of Investigation. (n.d.). Table 43. Retrieved July 9, 2021, from Fbi.gov website: https://ucr.fbi.gov/crime-in-the-u.s/2012/crime-in-the-u.s.-2012/tables/43tabledatadecoverviewpdf

TAHIT Public Service Announcement. (2010, August 18). Retrieved June 18, 2021, from https://www.youtube.com/watch?v=UBLuaoGXOBg

Taking action against clinician burnout: A Systems Approach to Professional Well-Being report release event - National Academy of Medicine. (2019, September 30). Retrieved June 1, 2021, from Nam.edu website: https://nam.edu/event/taking-action-against-clinician-burnout-a-systems-approach-to-professional-well-being-report-release-event/

Tamblyn, R., Abrahamowicz, M., Dauphinee, D., Wenghofer, E., Jacques, A., Klass, D., … Hanley, J. A. (2007). Physician scores on a national clinical skills examination as predictors of complaints to medical regulatory authorities. *JAMA: The Journal of the American Medical Association*, *298*(9), 993–1001.

Tamblyn, R., Abrahamowicz, M., Dauphinee, D., Wenghofer, E., Jacques, A., Klass, D., … Hanley, J. A. (2010). Influence of physicians' management and communication ability on patients' persistence with antihypertensive medication. *Archives of Internal Medicine*, *170*(12), 1064–1072.

Taylor, C., & Benger, J. R. (2004). Patient satisfaction in emergency medicine. *Emergency Medicine Journal: EMJ*, *21*(5), 528–532.

The IHI Triple Aim. (n.d.). Retrieved June 18, 2021, from Ihi.org website: http://www.ihi.org/Engage/Initiatives/TripleAim/Pages/default.aspx

Thomas, D. 24/7/365: The Evolution of Emergency Medicine [Motion Picture]. (2013).

Tompkins, D. A., Bigelow, G. E., Harrison, J. A., Johnson, R. E., Fudala, P. J., & Strain, E. C. (2009). Concurrent validation of the Clinical Opiate Withdrawal Scale (COWS) and single-item indices against the Clinical Institute Narcotic Assessment (CINA) opioid withdrawal instrument. *Drug and Alcohol Dependence*, *105*(1–2), 154–159.

Tookes, H., Bartholomew, T. S., Geary, S., Matthias, J., Poschman, K., Blackmore, C., … Spencer, E. (2020). Rapid identification and investigation of an HIV risk network among people who inject drugs -Miami, FL, 2018. *AIDS and Behavior*, *24*(1), 246–256.

Tsing, A. (2009). Supply chains and the human condition. *Rethinking Marxism*, *21*(2), 148–176.

Tsing, A. L. (2017). *The Mushroom at the End of the World: On the Possibility of Life in Capitalist Ruins*. Princeton, NJ: Princeton University Press.

Tyser, A. R., Abtahi, A. M., McFadden, M., & Presson, A. P. (2016). Evidence of non-response bias in the Press-Ganey patient satisfaction survey. *BMC Health Services Research*, *16*(1), 350. doi:10.1186/s12913-016-1595-z

UC Davis Department of Emergency Medicine. (n.d.). What to expect in the emergency department. Retrieved July 6, 2021, from Ucdavis.edu website: https://health.ucdavis.edu/emergency/Patient%20and%20visitor%20resources/20160628_what-to-expect.html

Underlying cause of death, 1999-2019 request. (n.d.). Retrieved July 9, 2021, from Cdc.gov website: https://wonder.cdc.gov/ucd-icd10.html

Understanding the epidemic. (2021, June 17). Retrieved July 7, 2021, from Cdc.gov website: https://www.cdc.gov/opioids/basics/epidemic.html

USFRI-University of South Florida. (n.d.). Policies & Procedures | USF. Retrieved June 18, 2021, from Usf.edu website: https://www.usf.edu/research-innovation/research-integrity-compliance/ric-programs/irb/hipaa/policies-procedures.aspx

Villalona et al. 2020. "Comments from Press-Ganey Survey Data January 1, 2012 – December 31, 2017." .American Journal of Emergency Medicine: 2743.

Villalona, S. (2018). *Looking Beyond Patient Satisfaction: Experiences of Spanish-Speaking Patients Seeking Non-Urgent* (University of South Florida). Retrieved from https://scholarcommons.usf.edu/cgi/viewcontent.cgi?article=8571&context=etd

Villalona, S., Boxtha, C., Webb, W. A., Cervantes, C., & Wilson, J. W. (2020a). "If at least the patient could not be forgotten about": Communication in the emergency department as a predictor of patient satisfaction. *Journal of Patient Experience*, *7*(6), 1015–1021.

Villalona, S., Cervantes, C., Boxtha, C., Webb, W. A., & Wilson, J. W. (2020b). "I Felt Invisible Most of the Time": Communication and satisfaction among patients treated in emergency department hallway beds. *The American Journal of Emergency Medicine*, *38*(12), 2742–2744.

Villalona, S., Jeannot, C., Yanez Yuncosa, M., Webb, W. A., Boxtha, C., & Wilson, J. W. (2020c). Minimizing variability in interpretation modality among

Spanish-speaking patients with limited English proficiency. *Hispanic Health Care International: The Official Journal of the National Association of Hispanic Nurses*, *18*(1), 32–39.

Vizient Inc. (n.d.). Retrieved June 19, 2021, from Vizientinc.com website: https://www.vizientinc.com/

Weiner, S. G., Baker, O., Bernson, D., & Schuur, J. D. (2020). One-year mortality of patients after emergency department treatment for nonfatal opioid overdose. *Annals of Emergency Medicine*, *75*(1), 13–17.

Welcome to Exeter Hospital Emergency Department. (2014, February). Retrieved July 6, 2021, from Exeterhospital.com website: https://www.exeterhospital.com/getmedia/4f513f96-2300-497b-86cd-1cdf0886ac4a/EHR_025_14-Emergency-Department-Fact-Sheet_1.pdf.aspx

Welcome to the Emergency Department. (2012, May). Retrieved July 6, 2021, from Yeovilhospital.co.uk website: https://yeovilhospital.co.uk/wp-content/uploads/2015/07/Welcome-to-the-Emergency-Department.pdf

Welcome to the...Emergency Department. (2011, July). Retrieved July 6, 2021, from NSW website: https://www.health.nsw.gov.au/Performance/Documents/ed-patient-brochure.pdf

Wesson, D. R., & Ling, W. (2003). The clinical opiate withdrawal scale (COWS). *Journal of Psychoactive Drugs*, *35*(2), 253–259.

Wilson, J. W., & Wein, D. A. (2009). *Boarding Times and Patient Safety: A Generalizable Quantitative Model. Abstract 183*. Retrieved from https://www.annemergmed.com/article/S0196-0644(10)00812-7/pdf

Wilson, Jason W., Baer, R. D., & Villalona, S. (2019). Patient shadowing: A useful research method, teaching tool, and approach to student professional development for premedical undergraduates. *Academic Medicine: Journal of the Association of American Medical Colleges*, *94*(11), 1722–1727.

Wintemute, G. J. (2015). The epidemiology of firearm violence in the twenty-first century United States. *Annual Review of Public Health*, *36*(1), 5–19.

Yasumaro, S., Silva, M., Andrighetti, M., de Lourdes Macoris, M., Mazine, C., & Winch, P. (1998). Community involvement in a dengue prevention project in Marilia, São Paulo state, Brazil. *Human Organization*, *57*(2), 209–214.

Young, R. E. (1981). The epistemic discourse of teachers: An ethnographic study. *Anthropology & Education Quarterly*, *12*(2), 122–144.

Zhou, R. A., Baicker, K., Taubman, S., & Finkelstein, A. N. (2017). The uninsured do not use the emergency department more-they use other care less. *Health Affairs (Project Hope)*, *36*(12), 2115–2122.

Zismer, D. (2019). Framework to gauge physician burnout. *Physician Leadership Journal. May/June*, 50–54.

Index

Note: Page numbers in *italics* refer to figures.

About the Authors

Jason W. Wilson, MD, MA, FACEP, is an Emergency Medicine (EM) physician, medical director, and medical anthropologist with an interest in developing patient-centered pathways that are medically efficacious but also consider structural and cultural forces in determining health inequities while reconsidering the role and position of the Emergency Department (ED). Currently, Dr. Wilson is crafting an ED-based opioid and HCV colocated treatment pathway and conducting patient-informed research on nonfatal gunshot wound injuries to craft public health interventions to decrease firearm violence. Dr. Wilson is an associate professor and serves as a core faculty member of the Division of EM, Department of Internal Medicine, Morsani College of Medicine at the University of South Florida (USF) where he also holds an affiliated faculty title in the Department of Anthropology and serves on the leadership board for the Center for Justice Research and Policy.

Roberta D. Baer is a professor in the Anthropology Department of the USF. She received her PhD from the University of Arizona in 1984. Her areas of current research include applied medical and nutritional anthropology, and issues related to refugee health and dietary adaptation. For the past seven years, she has been working with Wilson on projects integrating applied medical anthropology into not only clinical spaces but also the training of medical professionals.

About the Contributors

Emily Holbrook, MA, is a PhD Candidate in the Department of Anthropology at the University of South Florida (USF). Ms. Holbrook has served as the graduate student assistant for Dr. Wilson and Baer's undergraduate courses and is an expert at IRB compliance and protocol creation. Her PhD work is on healthcare access for refugees in the Tampa Bay Area.

Kilian Kelly, MA, completed his undergraduate BA in Anthropology at the USF. He was a student in the Physician-Patient Interaction course. Recently he completed an MA in Anthropology at Perdue.

Seiichi Villalona, MA, is a fourth-year medical student at the Rutgers Robert Wood Johnson Medical School in New Jersey. Mr. Villalona's MA thesis was completed in the Emergency Department (ED) at Tampa General and focused on issues of healthcare access for patients with limited English proficiency. While at USF, he also served as the graduate student assistant for Dr. Wilson and Baer's undergraduate courses and worked as a research assistant (RA) in the ED at Tampa General for three years.

Carlos Osorno-Cruz is a third-year medical student at the University of Iowa. He completed his undergraduate training at the USF. He was a student in the Patient-Physician Interaction undergraduate course and worked as a RA in the ED at Tampa General Hospital for two years.

Heather Henderson, MA, is a PhD Candidate in the Department of Anthropology at the USF. Ms. Henderson has served as the graduate student assistant for Dr. Wilson and Baer's undergraduate courses and has been instrumental in the design of patient-centered pathways for opioid use disorder.

www.ingramcontent.com/pod-product-compliance
Lightning Source LLC
Chambersburg PA
CBHW050650280326
41932CB00015B/2848